I AM Sex

I AM Sex

Dr. TaMara Griffin

ISBN: 151427034X
ISBN 13: 9781514270349

I AM Sex is grounded in more than 11 years of my academic research from studying women's beliefs, attitudes and behaviors regarding sexuality. It is also based on over 20 years of personal and professional experiences, stories from the beautiful women that I have worked with and counseled.

Dedication

This book is dedicated to my passion and my purpose!
Sex is who I AM! It flows through my veins! It's my heartbeat! I need it to breathe!!!

Acknowledgements and Thanks

FIRST AND FOREMOST, ALL GLORY and praises belong to the Most High! The Almighty! My Alpha and Omega, my Beginning and Ending and the The Author and The Finisher of my story- God! Thank you Father for blessing me and choosing me to share this powerful and life-saving message with your people. Father, I pray that you continue to use me and allow me to share this message of healthy sexuality until my very last breath. How dare I not? Father our people are perishing from a lack of knowledge. May the work that I do continue to be a blessing to the lives of others. Help them to understand the direct and indirect consequences of their sexual choices. Help them to understand the power and the responsibility of their sexuality. Lastly, Father help them to make safer and healthier informed decisions regarding their sexuality. In Jesus' name, Amen.

I would like to acknowledge and thank the following people for their unwavering support and encourage they have given me throughout the years. First and foremost, I would like to say thank you to my mother and father, Clarence and Bettina Campbell. When your 13 year old daughter said she wanted to be a sex therapist you did not shut her down, instead you helped her to make sense of what it really meant. I thank you for that! Daddy, no matter how much I talk about sex, I will always be your little girl! Momma, in so many ways I am just like you! And I would not have it any other way. You have taught me so much. I am so blessed to have you and daddy! Thank you for supporting and nurturing *all* my dreams. But most importantly, thank you for being praying parents and teaching me the importance of having a relationship with God.

I could not write a book about sexuality without thanking Dr. Caroline Yelding. Dr. Yelding, from the very first moment you walked into your Human Sexuality course at Alabama State University in the fall of 1993, as a wide-eyed and curious freshman, I was captivated! I remember thinking, I want to be just like her! You were the epitome of grace, beauty and sophistication. Thank you for taking me under your wing and becoming my mentor and role model. You may not realize how much of an impact you had on me but it is because of you that I became even more determined to pursue a career in human sexuality. So here I am, thank you!

I would like to thank Quan and Shanise Ollie for the amazing cover design. You guys rock! For the second time, you have captured my vision perfectly. It is always such a pleasure to work with you both. You have a gift. I pray that God increases your portion.

I have to thank my amazing editor FaLessia Booker! You did such an awesome job! Your comments and feedback helped to bring my dream to fruition! I could not have done it without you! You were invaluable and I thank you for the bottom of my heart!

am sending much love and many blessings to all the amazing men and women who have shared their personal stories with me. Thank you for entrusting me with the most sacred and vulnerable parts of your life! With all that I am, I thank you for all your support, encouragement and kind words over the years! It is because of you that I am able to do the work that I do. You inspire me! I honor, uplift, and thank you!

Last but not least, I thank my husband Marvin L. Griffin. Thank you Babe for understanding just how much this human sexuality thing means to me. Thank you for pushing me, even though sometimes I pushed back, to get my Doctorate degree in Human Sexuality and my Doctor of Philosophy in Human Sexuality! You love me unselfishly and unconditionally and for that, I am eternally grateful!

Table of Contents

Acknowledgements and Thanks · · · · · · · · · · · · · · · · · ix
Introduction · xiii
Chocolate · xvii
Down There! A Love Letter from Your Vagina · · · · · · xxvii

I AM Sex: Part One -Your Sexual Blueprint· ·1

Chapter 1:   Reclaiming Your Sexuality ·3
Chapter 2:   Designing Your Blueprint · 11

I AM Sex: Part Two - Understanding Your Sexuality · · · · · · · · · · · · 25

Chapter 3:   I AM Sex Trivia · 27
Chapter 4:   Why Women Have Sex · 29
Chapter 5:   Human Sexual Response Cycle · · · · · · · · · · · · · · · · · 35
Chapter 6:   Female Reproductive System· · · · · · · · · · · · · · · · · · · 44
Chapter 7:   Becoming Intimately Acquainted With Yourself· · · · · · ·58
Chapter 8:   The Menstrual Cycle, Pregnancy and Menopause · · · · ·63
Chapter 9:   Common Conditions of the Female
             Reproductive System · 73
Chapter 10: Sexually Transmitted Infections · · · · · · · · · · · · · · · · ·83

Chapter 11: How Can I Protect Myself From STIs? · · · · · · · · · · · · · ·98
Chapter 12: Routine Testing and Screenings Every
          Woman Should Have · 113
Chapter 13: Importance of Knowing Your Reproductive System · · · 120

I AM Sex: Part Three - I Am Ready for Pleasure · · · · · · · · · · · · · · 123

Chapter 14: You Are Now Ready! · 125
Chapter 15: Choreographing Your Sexual Pleasure · · · · · · · · · · · 127
Chapter 16: Intimacy Beyond Intercourse · · · · · · · · · · · · · · · · · 141
Chapter 17: Sexual Intercourse · 147
Chapter 18: Speaking of the BIG "O" · 153
Chapter 19: Communicating Your Sexual Desires? · · · · · · · · · · · · 161
Chapter 20: Sexperiment with Your Sexual Script! · · · · · · · · · · · 168
          Dr. TaMara Griffin Bio · 179
          Appendix A · 181

Introduction

Yes! I wanted to be A Sex Therapist At Age 13!

From the time I was 13, I wanted nothing more than to be a sex therapist.

"What?"

"Gasp!"

"What kind of parent lets their child say this?"

Some even clutch their pearls. These are just some of the typical responses I get when people read my bio without knowing me, hearing my story or learning about my journey into the field of human sexuality!

I grew up in a very "sex positive" environment: my mother was very open and honest when it came to sexuality. Sometimes, she was a little too open, but nevertheless, she made sure that my questions never went unanswered.

I was introduced to the field of human sexuality, via reproductive health, at a very early age. Many of the women in my family, including myself, suffered from reproductive health issues. Being exposed to their experiences as well as mine, I developed a natural curiosity about these conditions. Being very inquisitive at a young age, I asked a lot of questions. I wanted to understand what was going on in my body as well as theirs.

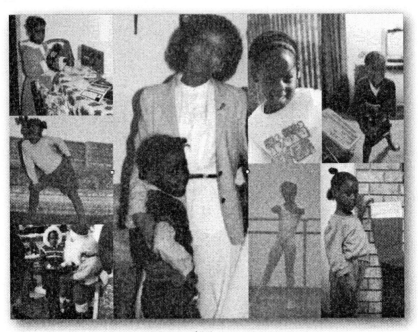

Me and Mom 1981

My mom was always very open and honest about sex! Sometimes maybe…just a little too much. But what I truly appreciate about my mom is that she never really held back.

Circa 1981, a nine year old girl is in her bedroom, sitting on her bed getting ready for sleep and playing with her baby dolls. This was a night I would never forget…little did I know that I would have a night that changed my life forever.

I was on my bed playing with my baby doll, minding my own business when my mom entered my room. In her hands were the purple Childcraft #15 Encyclopedia and a bag of "stuff" which I had never seen before. What could she want? Now I had already peeked in that book many times before, so I knew (with a very basic understanding) that that book was all about big kid "stuff." Why was she coming in my room with that book in her hand?

When she saw the perplexed look on my face, my mother must have sensed my confusion because she immediately stated that I had done nothing wrong. "I just want to talk to you about where babies come from." Immediately, I remembered that not too long ago, I had asked her this same question, and now my mom felt the need to answer. Equipped with all her armor, she began to explain.

As she talked about menstrual cycle, vaginas, wombs, maxi pads and belts, I stared in utter disgust. As if "the talk" wasn't bad enough, she had the nerve to demonstrate how to use that doggone belt! I remember thinking, "Enough already, enough!" All I wanted to do was play with my baby dolls.

From that initial conversation, I immediately began to have more questions! My mother would always answer my questions. In a very age- and developmentally-appropriate manner, she would talk with me about the female anatomy, physiology and various other aspects of sexuality. To convey her message in a way that I could understand, she would use things that were relevant to me like books, my favorite songs and even some of my favorite TV shows, like *90210* and *A Different World* to help educated me about all aspects of sexuality.

As my mother saw my interest in sexuality peaking, every so often, we would have conversations about sexuality. The topics would vary from what I learned in school, and included everything from crushes on the little boys in school to the media messages in songs and on the television. There was no internet back then.

One day, when I was 13, we were having a conversation about sexuality, but this particular conversation went a little differently and I actually think my mom was the one who was intrigued. The conversation went something like this:

"Momma, I've been thinking and I know what I want to be when I grow up!"

"Ok. What now? Let me guess….a singer." That was her guess because during that time, I loved to sing and I actually had a pretty good voice. And up until that moment, her answer would have been correct.

"No, not anymore. I want to be something else."

"Ok, you've changed your mind. What is it now?"

"A Sex Therapist!"

Silence. Blank stare. Blink.

"A what? A sex therapist? Where in the world did you get that from?" There was definitely a look of concerned curiosity on her face. But before she flew off the handle, she waited anxiously to hear my response and assess my true understanding of what I had just shared.

"Well, I want to help people learn about sex and talk about sex the way you talk to me and my friends. Some people do not have their mom to talk to and I want to help them by talking to them so they can learn too."

I remember my mom exhaling with a sigh of relief because my answer was based on my 13 year understanding of talking about sex. My answer was valid and it was not anything way off in left field. Nor was it anything of an inappropriate sexual nature. And of course, like a mother, she continued to probe until she was completely comfortable and sure of what I meant by wanting to be a sex therapist.

As I think back, I am not exactly sure where I learned the term "sex therapist," but in my mind there was nothing negative, nasty or taboo associated with the term. Even at that age in my life, all being a sex therapist mean to me was helping people talk about the sex the way my mother had talked to me.

Because my mother was such a sex positive person, she was determined to break the cycle and lack of education which she did not receive from my grandmother. She continued to empower my dream and educate me about sexuality. My mother helped to cultivate and nurture my passion by exposing me to resources such as Planned Parenthood's Peer Health Educators, which I eventually became a part of at age 16. As I spent time learning more about sexuality through my conversations with my mom, age-appropriate books and sex education classes in school, I knew I wanted to do with the rest of my life. Yes, at 13 I knew I wanted to be a sex therapist.

Chocolate

As I taste you, you melt like chocolate in my mouth and all over my hand
mouth-watering temptation so sweet
taunting, teasing and stimulating my tongue
I lick the seduction of your sweetness which merely entices me to want
to need......more
greedily, I indulge
filled until I am full
dripping, oozing with passion
I exhale
licking my lips full
full with satisfaction as I reach the pentacles of euphoria
I am drawn into you
chocolate, for I cannot resist
your chocolate
trembling with emotion
feigning for passion
can I please have a hit
just to think, this was only the first taste

Fast forward to age 16, a group of teenage girls on the way to the mall talking and giggling about the little mannish boys that we have crushes on. Yet again, mom decides it is the perfect opportunity to have "the talk!" Although I was embarrassed, I was still intrigued. I think her attempt to explain what the desire to have sex felt like was pretty interesting!

So here we are in this car, basically trapped, listening to my beloved mother talk about raging hormones, being horny and what it feels like to crave sex. I can still hear the conversation very clearly: "young ladies, you all are at the age where you're liking boys and your bodies are going to begin to starting having feelings and craving sex." Of course, one of my overzealous friends had to ask the question, "ooh, ooh—what does it feel like," raising her hand like we were in school.

Now all of us were on the edge of our seats, waiting to hear the response. My mother said…. "Craving sex is like the craving you have for chocolate." Now, I'm thinking, "chocolate, whew, that must be real good because I loooooooooove chocolate!" Then she went on to further explain that the way our body craves things we like is the same feeling—we will begin to want it all the time once we get a taste. It is the feeling that we have when we are horny. Horny? I could just shrivel up and die— oh the horror of your mom saying "horny!" Of course, she went on to explain further that although we have this craving, it's not necessarily always good for us because it can cause consequences that we were not ready for.

As I think back, what she said made perfect sense in my 16 year old mind because I absolutely loved chocolate and I could totally relate to that desire. I understood the consequences of eating too much chocolate. That conversation would be one of many that would linger in my mind and eventually add fuel to the passion of my interest in the field of human sexuality.

By the age of 16, I was a peer health educator with Planned Parenthood and I also had begun working at an agency with children whose parents were HIV positive. That experience was so invaluable.

The ability to touch the lives of those who were experiencing significant trauma and to be able to help them move forward despite the grief and loss further inspired me to continuing working in the field of human sexuality.

Although my mom was always sex positive and very open and honest about sexuality, there were definitely some things that she left out! I know you're probably thinking, "What in the heck could she have possibly left out?" She covered periods, pads, belts, bras, crushes, consequences and chocolate!

Well actually, there were a lot of things she left out… and I'm sort of glad she did, because I think talking about sexual positions that her and my dad used could have been very traumatic and ruined my images of sex forever. Even now….the visual…ugh, never mind!

Hey—that might actually be a great method of birth control for some kids! Imagine mom and dad walking in the rooms saying to their kids, "Hey! Your mom and I just some amazing sex! Wanna hear all about it?" I don't know about ya'll, but that might have just ruined everything for me!

Nevertheless, I'm very grateful for what she did tell me. I am more grateful what the things I learned on my own—orgasms, female ejaculation and sex toys—OH MY!!! Whew!!

Okay… bring it back!

So you see, for me leaning about sex was quite different than one might have expected. My initial introduction and education about sexuality was less focused on the physical dimension, but rather the other dimensions of sexuality. I learned about the direct and indirect consequences of sex. I also learned about the social determinants and the impact that they can have on sexuality. Learning about sex did not make me want to have sex—it had the opposite effect. Learning about sex empowered me to be able to make safer and informed decisions regarding sex so that when I was actually ready to have sex, I would be well prepared.

I was truly blessed to have a mother who talked to me about sex and was able to convey it in a way that made sense. I admired her so much so that she inspired me to want to talk to people and educate them in the same way that she educated me. Additionally, I did not want any woman to ever experience some of the things my family members and I had to undergo at the hands of physicians that lacked cultural humility and a thorough understanding of female reproductive health. Finally, I wanted to be a sex therapist at 13 years old because so many girls, including many of my friends, never had anyone to talk with them about sexuality. They did not even have basic information about their bodies, menstrual cycle, etc. The only message they received was "DON'T" because after all, sexuality is taboo, stigmatized, and something good girls don't do.

Now I know my experience was very unique! Many other young girls and even some women were not blessed enough to have someone to talk to about "the birds and the bees" and as a result, they were left to learn about sexuality from their friends, television, books, magazines or whatever they could get their hands on. Unfortunately, this lack of proper education and resources has helped to contribute to and even shape views regarding sexuality. In many ways, it is also the culprit behind the "down there" detachment or disassociation from our bodies which leads women to talk about our bodies as some separate entity apart from who we are. It also helps to contribute to the sexual dysfunction and negative and unhealthy ways in which we view our sexualities.

Furthermore, this lack of appropriate sex-positive information has left many women feeling sexually inadequate, misinformed and unprepared to have a sex-positive experience and positive sex-esteem, and may have caused them to put themselves at risk and/or in compromising situations and conform to some unhealthy sexual images that have been perpetuated by the media.

It was because of these experiences that I made it my mission to talk about sex—because I AM sex. I wanted to empower women and girls with the knowledge and skills and tools to make safer and healthier decisions regarding their sexuality. I wanted to teach them how to advocate for themselves so that they would not feel ashamed, embarrassed or belittled. I wanted them to love themselves and their bodies. I wanted them to celebrate their sexuality but most importantly, I wanted them to be proud of who they are as women. It is because of this that I devoted myself to empowering women to discover, explore, celebrate and embrace their sexual selves. My passion is deeply rooted in spreading messages of healthy sexuality, breaking intergenerational patterns that contribute to unhealthy and negative behaviors and changing images of women of hypersexualized in the media to create sex positive images.

My thoughts and definition of sex are probably a lot different than most authors, therapists, etc. I focus on sexuality from a comprehensive and holistic aspect. I focus on the entire person, their surroundings, social identities, environment, and everything outside of the bedroom in addition to the physical part that takes place inside the bedroom, car, airplane or wherever intercourse is happening. Please believe me when I say your life is your sexuality, and how you experience life in all its dimensions is how you will experience sexuality.

In this 40th year of my life, I am more than humbled and honored to say that I have been blessed to be able to do something that I truly love. It's not very often that someone can find something that completes them, but it's even more powerful when that something finds and becomes you—that is divine! I know that this is my passion, my purpose, my gift and my ministry and on the pages of this book, I share with you all that I am. Who am I? I am woman, I am a life, I am love, but most importantly *I AM Sex*!

I—LOVE—SEX!!

Yes, I do! Ok, now that I have your attention…yes! This is a book about just how much I love sex, but not necessarily in the context of what you may be thinking. And no—before you begin to wonder—it is not some sordid, twisted memoir of my personal clandestine sexcapades. However, it is a tell-all, fun, sexy and entertaining book containing all the wonderfully amazing things about sex, some of which your mother never told you—well, unless you had a mother like mine!

I AM Sex is an attempt to undo and dispel all the unhealthy and negative messages that women have received about sexuality over the years.

It's also designed to create a healthy sex-esteem and to give women permission to love sex just as much as I do!

I AM Sex is the culmination of my journey through the field of human sexuality over the past 24 years. On the pages of this book, you'll find educational information, questions and answers, sensual poetry, and "Pearls of Wisdom," which are my unique tips, tools and skills that will help you embrace your sexuality.

My lens on the spectrum of sexuality is very unique! I see beautiful shades and fluidity that blend together to customize and create our own individual sexual blueprint. It is with this blueprint that we build and shape our sexuality.

I AM Sex is that blueprint and on the pages of it, you shall find yourself. Whether you are a single mom, a married housewife, a college student or a professional working woman, there will be something on these pages for you. It doesn't matter whether you are a virgin, sexually experienced or sexually repressed—there is something on these pages for you. Black or white, yellow or green, there is something on these pages for you!

Word for word, sentence for sentence, page for page, I encourage you to open and expand your heart to receiving the message that is here for you. Hopefully this book will challenge you to learn things, to make different choices, to ask probing questions, and to take steps to fully celebrating and embracing your sexual self.

Allow me to share my most intimate self with you….because—I—AM—Sex!

"Have You Ever Stopped to Think about Just How Much Damage You've Actually Cost and/or Done To Your Sexual Self Over The Years?"
—Dr. TaMara

Down There! A Love Letter from Your Vagina

"Down there," "you know… that," "it," or "this area," are some of the vague or slang expressions we use when referring to our female anatomy. The sometimes awkward nature in which we talk about our vaginas gives the impression that it's some deep, dark, mysterious black hole or something. We are so embarrassed by and disconnected from our vaginas that that we don't even associate it as part of our own body. Why is that?

There are many reasons women disassociate themselves from owning the beauty of the vagina. In addition, the messages we receive from media, family, friends and even ourselves regarding women's vaginas are not always the most empowering. Some are even over-sexualized and downright degrading. Society perpetuates the belief that the vagina is this dirty thing that needs to be cleansed of its filth, as evident by all the feminine hygiene products on the market. There are even cosmetic procedures to "pretty up" the ugly, disgusting vagina. Constantly being inundated with such messages, how does one not hold a shameful view of the vagina? It's beliefs, attitudes and feelings like these that contribute to the unhealthy behaviors that put women at risk for HIV and other sexually transmitted infections, victimization, abuse, body image issues, unhealthy relationships, mental health challenges and so much more.

When was the last time you grabbed a mirror and looked at your vulva; touching and exploring its delicate and intricate folds? How many times have we actually taken the opportunity to get to know our vagina? If you could have a conversation with your vagina, what would she say? Would it be a reunion between happy old friends or a bittersweet greeting of strangers on the street? Would there be an exchange of pleasantries or apologies? If another one of your friends happened to walk in on the conversation, would you be embarrassed to introduce her or would you be proud of her feminine power and beauty? If she asked you the question, can you honestly say you took good care of her all these years? Or would she burst into tears because you disassociate yourself from her because of the fear, shame, stigma, judgment, trauma and disrespect you allowed her to endure from others?

It's time for a shift. We must begin to break those negative intergenerational patterns and disempowering media messages that contribute to a lack of SEX-esteem when it comes to our genitalia. Just as no two women are alike, no two vulvas and vaginas are alike; they are just as unique as each of us! It's important to become intimately acquainted with our bodies. Not just the correct terminology and function, but also understanding the power and connection to all the dimensions of sexuality. We must to learn to value, embrace, honor and celebrate all of our womanhood, for our vagina is the door of life and also a means of providing pleasure. How could we not respect its power, purpose and beauty?

Apologize this moment for any lack of respect, love and appreciation! It is time to make things right and allow her to reclaim her rightful place right now!

I AM Sex: Part One - Your Sexual Blueprint

Reclaiming Your Sexuality

How do we move toward reclaiming our sexuality? By first loving ourselves, understanding that we are sexual beings, and giving ourselves permission to discover, explore, unleash, celebrate, embrace and honor our sexuality. Women's sexuality is far more powerful than we can ever imagine. Tapping into and honoring the power is fundamental to the journey.

As women, we are becoming more empowered and proactive in managing our sexuality by learning to accept, embrace and celebrate our sexual selves by redefining who we are as sexual beings. In the past, biology, gender roles, sexual norms, and a history of negative intergenerational patterns have put women at greater risk of HIV/AIDS and other sexually transmitted infections. Many women have received insufficient information about sexuality and sexual behaviors, making them vulnerable and powerless to protect themselves. This misinformation, along with stigma, label and judgment have made it difficult for women to enjoy and appreciate their sexuality. It's time to transform judgment into love, do away with labels, dispel myths and start replacing them with messages of empowerment.

So how do we begin to embrace our sexual selves? It's time to reclaim the number one spot in our lives. Loving ourselves first has to become the priority! We must embrace and understand the power we possess, simply because we are women! Knowing how and when to use that power is all a part of redefining our sexuality. We must become

Sexperts! Learning to become intimately acquainted with ourselves and understanding our body is essential to having power over of our sexuality. Additionally, learning to understand, respect and communicate our sexual attitudes, beliefs, needs, wants and concerns, not only to our physicians, but our mates, is imperative in helping to navigate healthier relationships and safer and more satisfying sexual experiences.

Building self-acceptance, self-esteem and self-efficacy and maintaining self-care are the steps to embracing our sexual selves. We must learn to love and accept ourselves, flaws and all. By doing so, we begin to free ourselves from the confines of judgment and scrutiny of others, thus giving ourselves permission to discover, explore & unleash our feminine powers!

Self-Acceptance. To thine ownself be true! In order to love yourself, you must be true to who you are! This can be achieved by embracing and honoring who you are and where you are at this very moment in time. Self-acceptance also means understanding that you are not perfect and knowing that's ok. Beauty is not defined by perfection, but character. However, if you find something within your character to be unfitting, self-acceptance empowers you to actively seek out ways to improve that which you find unfitting. It also gives you the strength to change. And during this time of transition and growth, self-acceptance allows you to find peace and appreciation within the process because self-acceptance understands that it's not about the destination, but rather the journey.

Self-Esteem. Self-esteem is powered by self-acceptance. Once you can accept yourself you can begin to love yourself, flaws and all! When you are operating from a high level of self-esteem, you are less likely to put yourself in harm's way and more likely to take care of yourself. You do not allow your integrity, dignity, safety or health to become comprised. A woman of distinction, yet meek and humble in character; your reputation does not become you. You do not allow others to define you:

"If you don't define yourself for yourself, you'll be crunched into other people's fantasies of you and eaten alive."—Audrey Lorde

Self-Efficacy. In addition to having high self-esteem, high self-efficacy is an essential element of loving yourself first. Self-efficacy is a belief in your ability to succeed in any given situation. Your sense of self-efficacy plays a major role in how you set goals, approach tasks, handled challenges and overcome obstacles. A woman with high self-efficacy believes that she can do whatever she puts her mind to. Even if she doesn't know how to do something, she has enough dignity to ask, without feeling threatened or losing sight of who she is and her capability. However, she realizes there is strength in vulnerability and uses it as a platform to success. She utilizes her talents and gifts for a purpose beyond herself.

Self-Care. The intention of self-care lies in its focus on preventative care versus treatment. Self-care is essential in embracing your sexuality. Operating from a place of self-love includes maintaining balance within the 10 Sexual Dimensions of Wellness: mental, emotional, spiritual, social, legal, economic, chemical, energetical, political, institutional and physical.

Mental—As you read earlier in the book, it can be difficult to stop thinking about sex—after all, the brain is the biggest sex organ! Thanks to the brain, certain hormones help to regulate and control our sexual desires, attractions and how we love. Keep in mind that the body and brain remember great sexual experiences. Those experiences get imprinted into cell memory, making it difficult to get over things and move on. Furthermore, chemicals and hormones also impact our emotional stability.

Emotional—Sex inevitably creates an emotional connection. The emotional consequences of sex can have long lasting effects. Emotional consequences can encourage an individual to make decisions that he or she would not normally make. The fluctuation of the chemicals and hormones in our brain keep us wanting sex and coming back for more and more. In addition, emotional consequences may include the inability of a person to form strong emotional bonds of love, intimacy, attachment and/or trust.

Spiritual—Reconciling your spirituality, faith and/or beliefs with your sexual desires and response is essential to maintaining sexual self-care. For people who may be practicing abstinence, celibacy or who were raised to believe that sex before marriage is wrong, a slip-up of engaging in sex may cause them to question their morals and values, which is not only spiritually conflicting, but emotionally draining. Another important fact to keep in mind is that every time you have sex with someone, you are having sex with everyone that they had sex with as well and that energy, and sometimes STIs, transfers from person to person. Therefore, it is extremely important to consider the spiritual ramifications of sex.

Social—Often, people who engage in casual sex, especially women, develop a negative reputation which can leave you socially destroyed. This reputation has a tendency to follow you and even may prevent someone from taking you seriously or seeing you as "relationship material." Additionally, if one or both parties are married, the havoc on the spouse(s) and any children involved can be very detrimental and leave a lasting negative impact on all parties involved.

Legal—You have fallen victim to your hormones and you are now a "friend of the court." The process of establishing paternity can be frustrating and takes an emotional toll on everyone involved. Now you must deal with potentially missing work, late child support payments, garnishment, legal fees, and destroyed relationships, all because you were blinded by sex. Unfortunately, many times the one who is truly the casualty of this one-night stand is the child because the parents cannot seem to work things out in a mature manner.

Economic—In a moment of passion, for whatever reason, you fail to practice safer sex. As a result, you end up pregnant, getting someone pregnant or get infected with a sexually transmitted infection. Now, you are paying for treatment of an STI or child support, dealing with court costs, and time off work.

Chemical—With all of the ups, downs and hormonal shifts happening during attraction, sexual arousal, ejaculation and orgasm, it is important that we learn how to be aware of them and find balance. Without any awareness of neurochemistry and how it can wreak havoc on our lives and relationship, we continuously put ourselves at risk for unintended consequences of sexuality. However, when we are aware of these shifts, we are better prepared to make healthier and informed decisions regarding our sexual health.

Energetical—When two people have sex, there is an exchange of energy. Hormones are released into the bloodstream that help to bond people together. In addition, when it comes to sexual intercourse, the receiving partner literally receives something inside of their body. Given the fact that sex, casual or not, involves an intimate exchange of energy, one should take into consideration the ramifications of engaging in the horizontal mambo. Learning to protect your energy is essential! Your energy is the vitality of life. Allowing someone to negatively impact your energy will ultimately drain you of your power.

Political—The political fallout and ramifications of sex can be devastating and leave lasting effects on the individual, their family and the community. Political belief systems and agendas have a major influence on how sexuality is constructed and viewed in society.

Depending on the political climate, prioritizing funding for sexual health programs, care and treatment can be limited. In such cases, political decisions limit access to health care, treatment, and programs, especially for those who are in a lower socioeconomic status and/or depending on government programs to provide health care insurance. Political agendas can also promote reproductive justice and advocacy for issues such as determining the "freedom" that organizations have in providing reproductive health care services to employees, abstinence versus comprehensive sex education curricula in schools and same-sex marriage and equality rights.

Institutional—Institutions such as faith-based organizations, hospitals, universities and colleges can serve as a protective factor or risk factor for sexuality, depending on the context in which sexuality is defined by a particular institution. Institutions that create an open, safe, non-judgmental space for conversations about healthy sexuality help to serve as protective factors, whereas institutions that demonize sexual thoughts, beliefs, behaviors and attitudes serve as a risk factor for sexuality by continuing to further stigmatize sexuality.

Physical—There is always the risk of sexually transmitted infections, HIV and unintended pregnancy whenever a person has sex. Even though condoms and dental dams are considered effective when used consistently and correctly, there is always a chance for failure, especially if there is alcohol or some other substance involved. In addition, if there has been multiple casual sexual encounters with the same person, comfort levels begin to disappear and so does the likelihood of using a condom. The question you must ultimately as yourself is, "Is this one casual encounter worth the consequence and repercussions that might follow?"

Reframing sexuality as who we are versus something that we do will also help us begin to embrace our sexual selves.

Additionally, we must begin to dispel myths, tackle taboos and break the negative cycles of inter-generational patterns by redefining of views of sexuality and begin to accept it as something that is a natural, beautiful way of life. We were created as sexual beings with the gift to bring forth life. Understanding this miracle, our responsibility and the role of who we are with the spectrum of sexuality will allow us to continue to birth powerful changes into our lives and the lives of those with whom we come in contact with, ultimately changing the world one person at a time.

Inside each and every woman lives a beautiful, sensual, exotic woman yearning to reveal herself for all to behold and marvel at the mere essence of her phenomenon. Allow yourself to discover, explore and unleash your unique and individual feminine powers.

"We need to take a more proactive role in managing our sexual experiences by learning to accept, embrace and celebrate our sexual selves and by redefining who we are as sexual beings".—Dr. TaMara

Understanding your sexuality and the impact on life is part of your creating and/or revising your sexual blueprint, which is also a part of reclaiming your sexuality. Women have a very complex relationship with sexuality that contributes to the disempowerment of our sexuality and the denial of our sexual pleasure, wants, needs and desires.

Unhealthy and negative beliefs, thoughts and images of sexuality continuously bombard us on a daily basis. Sex is visible in all forms of media from party ads, club flyers, television, music and videos. Although music and videos are influential in impacting the sexuality of women and girls, televisions shows also play a significant role. TV programs such as *The Real Housewives* and *The Bachelorette* are filled with the same old script: images unhealthy relationships, lack of sisterhood, a false sense of self-esteem, overt sexual undertones and are famous for promoting "status" and "using what you got to get what you want." These TV shows and many others help to further contribute to the unhealthy images of women and girls. In addition, they help to add to the layers of intergenerational patterns, stigma, shame, guilt and embarrassment surrounding sexuality. Unfortunately, women have become so desensitized to seeing themselves being portrayed negatively that these images have become the norm for societal standards. While there aren't any signs that these unhealthy and demeaning images will disappear any time soon, there is definitely a need to counteract them. We are in need of a new sexual blueprint of empowerment, one which restores the dignity and character of women and girls.

Designing Your Blueprint

SEXUAL EMPOWERMENT

We have allowed the media to capitalize on our sexuality as if we were nothing more than objectified erotic capital. We are so busy trying to prove to everyone that we are so sexually empowered that we are actually doing ourselves a huge disservice. In many ways, the sexual behaviors that represent us in the media place us on the auction block for sale and for the entertainment of others— and we have the audacity to call this sexual empowerment?

Given the historical context and social construction of women's sexuality, it's important to move forward and reclaim and redefine images in the name of sexual empowerment in a way that does not cause us to compromise our integrity, and rejects negative stereotypes and media messages regarding hyper-sexualized, out of control women.

I'm all for sexual empowerment of women—however, within that empowerment comes a responsibility! It's not to be taken lightly. Being sexually empowered does not necessarily equate to engaging in sexual trysts all willy-nilly, nor does it mean gyrating, grinding and "twerking" all over the place!

It's my body and I'm free to do with it what I want and express my sexuality however I choose is the mantra of many sex positive feminist who revel in disdain for anyone who feels differently or expresses another view of sexual empowerment. To them I reply, "yes, why certainly is, but that 'freedom' does not come without a cost." Yes, you are free to engage in sexual expressions of all kinds, and yes, it is your body...nevertheless, there is a price to pay! That price that we pay comes in various forms such as: embodying all the negative energy exchanged from the sexual escapades, the negative impressions and unwanted attention, the messages that our young girls receive, sexual transmitted infections. In addition, this price we pay adds to the reasons why women continue to be disenfranchised, sold as a commodities and continue to remain as on bottom in every area from careers, educations, marriage, etc. Some will say, "sex sells" and "we use what we got to get what we want." And I absolutely agree...however, my question would be, "Is what we're getting worth what we're selling or giving away for free?"

The essence of sexual empowerment does not lie in the ability to make yourself orgasm! It's so much more than twerking! And it's beyond casual sexual encounters and one night stands, for we are more than our bodies!

Sexual empowerment is an emotional, mental, spiritual, social, legal, economic, chemical, energetical, political, institutional and physical accountability of our sexuality. Sexual empowerment is also about choice. That choice can be a decision to be sexual, but it can also be a decision to *not* be sexual. It is the choice that matters; the ability to freely decide which option is best for us on our own terms, without pressure or coercion from outside forces.

Sexual empowerment is about loving oneself unconditionally, flaws and all. It is about being wise about whom we share our energy with, understanding the unintended consequences of our indiscretions and realizing our worth and value beyond the bedroom.

Sexual empowerment is all about knowing and understanding our bodies, the parts and how they function. It is about advocating for access to reproductive healthcare. Our bodies bring forth life and LIFE! This is a crucial part of our sexual responsibility and one that should not be taken lightly! We nurture the world in our womb, therefore how can be bring forth healthy generations with worn and rotten wombs from poor choices of our past? How can we educate our girls when we have no real concept of sexual empowerment? We can't—as a result, we fail our generation and perpetuate the cycle of this false sense of sexual empowerment.

I challenge you to evaluate your assumptions on sexual empowerment! Wrap your mind around the damage that has been created by the miseducation of a generation. Push yourselves to move past the societal conceptualization of women's sexualities and move past our current thoughts of sexual empowerment. When we can truly create a sexual blueprint for women's sexuality, that can be authentically empowering.

BARRIERS TO SEXUAL EMPOWERMENT

Understanding past influences—childhood, past relationships, baggage, experiences, culture, race, ethnicity, gender—are critical, because these things are embedded into our sexual blueprints.

In order to begin this journey to sexual empowerment, you first have to understand what is blocking your path. You must identify obstacles to sexual empowerment that are hidden deep within your subconscious. It is time to identify those obstacles so that you can consciously and actively deal with them.

How do we do this?

This process begins by first taking an honest look into the very depths of our souls to understand our context of sexuality, who we are as sexual beings, and those intrinsic and extrinsic influences. We also must factor in our cultural, gender, social, religious and spiritual values, morals and sexual thoughts, beliefs and behaviors and the role each plays in helping to shape our sex-esteem. Moreover, we must understand how all of this shows up within the Dimensions of Sexuality. All of these things are embedded within our sexual blueprint. Peeling back these layers is critical to overcoming obstacles and becoming sexually empowered.

"Figure out who you are separate from your family, and the man or woman you're in a relationship with. Find who you are in this world and what you need to feel good alone. I think that's the most important thing in life. Find a sense of self because with that, you can do anything else." — Angelina Jolie, *Cosmopolitan Magazine*

INTERGENERATIONAL/CROSS-GENERATIONAL PATTERNS

Passed down from generation to generation, unhealthy negative patterns, behaviors and beliefs are like viruses replicating and spreading from one family member to another, infecting our thought patterns and becoming deep-rooted within the subconscious mind.

As young girls, we learned about ourselves from what we were taught and exposed to (or not exposed to) by our mothers, who learned from her mother, who learned from her mother and so on. If our mother did not know how to be empowered, it would have been next to impossible for her to teach her daughter how to be an empowered woman. This is not an attempt to place blame on mothers for anything, but rather to help identify some of the behavior patterns that may contribute to the very circumstances you face today. And because you haven't been taught and don't know any differently, you will continue to make the same mistake until you identify the dangerous, negative cyclical behaviors and commit to changing them.

"You are much more powerful today than the old thoughts, beliefs and behaviors that were programmed and absorbed during your childhood." — Wayne Dyer

You are not obligated to fulfill the destiny dictated to you through kinship. You can decide at this very moment to break the negative cycle by reprogramming your thoughts, beliefs and behaviors. By doing so, you begin to chart a new course, you can change destiny yourself as well as for future generations of women within your family.

Give yourself permission to identify each old negative pattern, behavior and/or belief; examine it; make peace with it; and release it to the universe as your first step towards empowerment/healing.

LOW SELF-ESTEEM

The gateway to disempowerment and low self-esteem can be an obstacle to loving ourselves. If we don't love, or even like, ourselves, how can we believe that we deserve better? How could we ever position ourselves for greatness? We can't!

When we lack self-esteem, we tend to place ourselves at risk because we don't care enough to believe we can do any better. Low self-esteem usually manifests itself in self-defeating behaviors, lack of confidence and lack of trust in oneself—all blocks to becoming and living an empowered lifestyle. When we lack self-esteem, we allow ourselves to be used and abused, seeking that which we believe is missing. Alternatively, we find comfort in sex, drugs, risky behaviors and other unhealthy compulsions.

Another effect of low self-esteem is a false sense of self with a super inflated self-esteem. In this case, we fool ourselves into believing that we have high self-esteem, when in actuality it is just over compensating for that which we lack or disapprove of. To protect ourselves, or in an effort to seek approval from the outside world, we create images and schemes of grandeur to "keep up" or to "fit it." Because we fear that our peers and/ or loved ones may find an unacceptable trait, disapprove or find us less than desirable, we become this "character" in an effort to divert their attention from finding out who we really are. However, when we become someone or something other than who we are, we are no longer true to ourselves. There begins the battle of duality between the true self and the ego because we have, in essence, said that who we are is not good enough so we create an alternate reality in an effort to be "loved."

"You find love in quotation marks here because when someone truly loves you, they accept you just as you are at that very moment, without conditions, limitations or faultfinding." — Unknown

When you truly love yourself, you think enough of yourself not to place yourself in harm's way. You think enough of yourself to put yourself first. You think enough of yourself to know that you deserve the best and accept nothing less!

LACK OF DECISION MAKING SKILLS

"A double minded man is unstable in all his ways." - James 1:8, *Bible*

Decision making is an essential part of life. Every decision we make has the propensity to affect our life—positively or negatively—which is why it is essential to develop healthy decision making skills.

Often the causes of indecisiveness or lack of proper decision making skills are more mental than physical and are deep rooted in the mind as a result of low self-esteem, low self-efficacy, bad relationships, poor self-image, a history of abuse, stress, and other factors.

"No perfect decision exists. Going back and forth can block you from going ahead." When you decide to take a risk, you get better at the process and learn what happens when you make leaps. Confidence grows with action."
— Steve Mensing

The art of decision making lies in our ability to make a balanced decision with minimal risk and maximized opportunity for growth. Because much of life hinges on the capacity to make safe, sound decisions, the inability to make rational decisions may have a much more profound impact our lives, making us more susceptible to engaging in unhealthy risky behaviors.

Common sense, wisdom, experience, confidence and trust in ourselves is what empowers us to make responsible decisions. If we do not make decisions, we cannot have our wants and/or needs met, have rewarding experiences or have vitally enriching lives. To live fully, we must embrace decisions with open hearts as an opportunity for growth. We must be willing to move beyond fear to empowerment by learning to trust in our ability to make healthier decisions.

LACK OF COMMUNICATION SKILLS

Communication involves the sharing and exchanging of information via verbal methods such as talking, listening, negotiating, compromising and non-verbal methods, such as body language.

The essence of relationships is communication; the lack of communication skills can seriously hinder those relationships. Lack of communication skills not only can damage your intimate personal relationships, but it can affect performance at work, self-confidence and even physical health.

When we experience problems in our relationships due to a lack of communication skills, we inappropriately attempt to share our feelings, and we may ultimately experience even more rejection, hurt, and misunderstanding. This may result in avoiding intimate communication and putting up emotional walls. When we cannot put our feelings into words, we often stare helplessly across an abyss of silence, or in frustration, hurl attacks that drive us further apart.

For any communication to be successful, the meaning that you wanted to convey must be understood. We must be assertive, honest and loving. Effective communication skills allows us to rebuild intimacy, understanding and clarity within relationships, thus removing the alienation and estrangement that may be felt as a result of not being able to communicate thoughts, feelings and beliefs.

SELF-DEFEATING THOUGHTS

"The most common way people give up their power is by thinking they don't have any." —Alice Walker

Resentment, guilt, criticism and fear: many of us carry around layers of negativity as a result of incidents that occurred in our past. We have built up layers that must be peeled in order to reach our core—our authentic self. We must begin to realize that we ultimately have control over our thoughts. We are responsible for the outcome of our experiences. We must begin to take ownership. If we continue to choose to believe that we are helpless victims, then the universe will continue to support us in that belief by drawing negative experiences to us. Once we begin to accept responsibility for our thoughts and behaviors, we free ourselves to change our thoughts and positive energy towards us.

"Facing the truth about yourself is vital to experience an empowering breakthrough to change and winning victory over self-defeating behaviors."— Dr. TaMara

DEATH WITH WORDS

A wise person once said, *"There are two things you can't take back, words and a speeding bullet."* Once either has been released into the universe, there is great potential for death. It is so important to think before you speak and to choose your words wisely. If there is nothing I have learned over the years, is that there is truly the power of life and death in the tongue. We have the ability to speak success or defeat over our lives, just based on the words we choose. If we choose to speak hate, we inadvertently bring more hate to our lives, just as if we speak love into lives, we'll experience more love. Hurtful words linger on in our mind, affecting our ability to make healthy decisions, thus putting us at increasing risk. When we have been told something over and over again, it eventually becomes our reality! It becomes who we are. And once these things become part of our subconscious and consciousness, we begin to manifest a death of our spirit by words.

Think about how many times you've been told, "you're this" or "you're that," "you're not good enough" or "smart enough." Initially, you may have not given in to this negativity; however, if this is something that has been continuously repeated over and over, eventually you may start to think, "Hey, maybe there is some truth to this." It's at that point that you begin to doubt yourself and eventually spiral into a negative pattern of unhealthy behaviors.

It is so important to affirm your worth on a daily basis! Start by facing yourself in the mirror and quoting positive affirmations. Tell yourself how beautiful you are—how you deserve nothing but the absolute best. Build yourself up, several times a day if needed. Soon you'll begin to believe what you are saying about yourself.

"We do not attract that which we want but that which we are." — Author James Allen

LACK OF SEX EDUCATION

In a day and age where HIV is still deadly, gonorrhea has resistant strains, celebrity sex tapes are the norm, sex sells everything, and casual sex is glamorized, we cannot afford to avoid the conversations about sex. We live in a time where technology makes everything accessible. With the click of a button, we can find out any and everything about sex; unfortunately, oftentimes the information is inaccurate, misleading and confusing.

Comprehensive sex education teaches the facts, dispels myths, removes the stigma and addresses taboos. Technology makes it possible for us to learn about sex from a variety of sources, many of which are not credible and do not offer information from an accurate educational standpoint. It's so important to provide the facts from a credible source like a credentialed sexologist, sex therapist, counselor or educator and not the internet or media.

We must get beyond the belief that comprehensive sex education equates to conversations about intercourse, different sexual positions, taking birth control, and having abortions. While some of those things are certainly a part of sex education, that is not the focal point of it. True comprehensive sex education includes conversations about the mental, emotional, spiritual, biochemical, social, legal, cultural and economic unintended consequences of sex—protected or unprotected. It also addresses how media messages impact sexuality and so much more.

We also must educate ourselves on personal responsibility and what it means to be accountable! We are in charge of our sexual health! We cannot rely on anyone else to make decisions regarding our sexual health. Failure to advocate and protect ourselves is like allowing ourselves to walk blindly into harm's way. Every time we have unprotected sex with someone whose HIV or sexually transmitted infection (STI) status we do not know, we are saying to them, "I love you enough to let you kill me!"

In addition to increasing knowledge, we must also increase skills! For example, it is not enough to teach that condoms prevent pregnancy and/or STIs—we must learn how to use a condom, how to negotiate condom usage with a partner, how to communicate safer sex options and even where to purchase and how to store condoms. Skills are essential! We can have all the knowledge and wherewithal in the world, but if we do not have the skills, then it is still an epic failure.

Understanding how our self-esteem, self-efficacy, triggers, social determinants (i.e., income, lack of insurance, poverty, lack of access to medical care, culture, religious beliefs, race, etc.) risk factors, strength factors and protective factors impact sexuality is important as well. Gaining an understanding of this may help to determine and/or shape the impact of our choices, beliefs, behaviors and attitudes on sexuality. In addition, it may help to reduce engaging in behaviors that puts oneself at risk for engaging in sexual behaviors that contribute, directly and indirectly, to the transmission of HIV and other STIs.

LACK OF KNOWLEDGE

"A people without knowledge shall perish." — *Bible*

"Ignorance is bliss" is the mantra of so many disempowered women, implying that some people would rather stay in a state of ignorance (lack of knowledge), than to face truth (educate themselves). Because the truth is so difficult for some people to deal with, they would rather not know—however, a lack of knowledge can prove to be just as hurtful.

When we lack knowledge, we find ourselves in compromising positions because we have failed to educate ourselves properly. And how can we make an effective and informed decision missing some of the pieces that complete the puzzle? Lack of knowledge leaves us in a weakened and impoverished condition which is not conducive to growth and empowerment.

"Knowledge itself is power." — Francis Bacon

The acquisition of knowledge is to enable the development of the mind as we strive to learn and understand our highest self. Our actions and movement then become a true manifestation of the Divine. Operating within the uniqueness of our highest self allows us to better understand others and our environment. Once you possess the knowledge of self, you become more empowered. However, with knowledge comes responsibility—the responsibility to do better, because now you know better.

Knowledge provides a beautiful blend of common sense and wisdom. Common sense is sound judgment and wisdom is the ability to discern the judgment and select the right course of action. When we tap into our knowledge base using our common sense and wisdom, we are more likely to make healthier and informed decisions that impact our lives in a positive way.

As girls, we are young and impressionable. We lack the knowledge and wisdom to discern. However, as we become adults, we gain the knowledge to make choices and change that which we deem unfitting.

"One of the greatest beauties of life is that we grow into wisdom and maturity from the knowledge we gain from our failures which in turn builds our greatest most empowered self." - Dr. TaMara

Overcoming Barriers

The road to sexual empowerment is paved with gold...NOT!!! If it were so, we all would be there—rich with happiness, peace of mind and lots of orgasms. But since it's not, then we must be willing to go the extra mile for the journey.

I don't think that change is truly something that you can ever be 100% ready for. Just as with seasons and time, change is inevitable and it is something that we all must go through at some point in our lives. On some level, you must be ready to change, or perhaps you picked up this book in hopes of learning something about your sexuality.

I encourage you to see this journey as an adventure. By opening your heart and mind and by changing your beliefs, you change who you are and you change the world around you.

Given the obstacles to sexual empowerment which may affect us to varying degrees, how do we move toward becoming sexually empowered? How do we remove the obstacles? How do we navigate the process?

Empowering change happens when you stay focused on your set of beliefs and you begin to align yourself with the same kind of energy. You are what you attract, not what you want. Additionally, in order for empowering change to occur, there must be a process of action and movement.

It begins with a shift in your consciousness thought patterns by removing self-defeating behaviors, negative cyclical patterns or other obstacles to empowerment and replacing them with an "I can" and " I will" attitude! You might be thinking that this sounds too good to be true. But I challenge you to wrap your mind around the "Empowered Consciousness Paradigm" (ECP) way of life: *faith (belief) + action (perseverance) + movement (patience) = the life you so desire*. Once you begin to embrace this powerful truth, no longer can you walk around with your eyes wide shut, for you are now privy to the secret to empowering change.

Faith is your belief in your ability. It's a system by which you live and believe.

<u>Action</u> is something can be done immediately. Without perseverance, there is no action.

<u>Movement</u> is a process happens over time. The word process here implies growth as a result of continuous ongoing practice.

Faith is the seed. Actions start the process of change, but without ongoing practice and perseverance, action cannot create enough momentum for real movement—that only happens over time with patience.

By committing yourself to following the "Empowered Consciousness Paradigm" way of life, you are one step closer to living the life you so desire! The ECP will help you incorporate small steps into your daily life so you are less likely to revert back to old behaviors and patterns. So no matter what your previous unhealthy behaviors, the guidance and steps offered within Empowered Consciousness Paradigm can help motivate you to improve not only your current state of sexuality, but your overall state of wellness. If you would like to learn more about the Empowered Consciousness Paradigm, I encourage you to pick up a copy of my best-selling book, *Live Inspired Feel Empowered (L.I.F.E.)*

Part of making lifestyle changes requires adopting new behaviors and changing how you live. But what we sometimes forget is that changing everything at once can be so overwhelming that we end up reverting back to old behaviors. Change can be difficult or easy depending upon how you view the process. Recognize that there may be a transitional period between the old and new behaviors and you may vacillate between your former behavior and thinking patterns, but don't be discouraged. This is normal when making any behavior change. I encourage you to set benchmarks for progress, acknowledge every effort you make and be gentle and loving to yourself along the way.

Ownership is the key to sexual empowerment. You have to really dig deep inside your soul to truly own it. You must face fears, dispel myths, negative intergenerational patterns and stigma about sexuality that society deems as acceptable. You must be willing to go against the status quo and become comfortable walking in your own heels.

The key to ownership is learning to accept and love yourself in all your colors—yes, even the part that you desire to change. Learning to trust and follow the divine spirit within yourself will enable you to find the strength and courage to own all that is authentically yours. As you begin to embrace the divine spirit within you, you will possess the capacity to manifest and attract all your sexual desires, wants, needs and/or beliefs; and that, my beloved, is true sexual empowerment!

As you begin to live this, your sexual truth, then it becomes easier to develop your empowered sexual consciousness.

"When the pupil is ready, the teacher will appear."— Unknown

I AM Sex: Part Two - Understanding Your Sexuality

I AM Sex Trivia

ARE THESE STATEMENTS TRUE OR FALSE? (See Appendix A for correct answers)

1. Sexual intercourse is the first sexual activity for females.
2. Self-Pleasure has always been recognized as normal sexual behavior.
3. All orgasms are the same.
4. Exercising can increase sexual pleasure and orgasmic intensity.
5. 95% of women DO NOT experience orgasm through self-pleasure.
6. The majority of women need direct clitoral stimulation to reach orgasm.
7. Self-Pleasure is often prescribed for pre-orgasmic women.
8. Stimulating the G-spot can cause female ejaculation.
9. The clitoris is made of erectile tissue.
10. There is a difference between arousal and desire.
11. Vibrators were first prescribed to treat hysteria in women.
12. Body image and sexuality are closely related.
13. Self-esteem and sexuality are closely related.
14. Women can experience a variety of different types of orgasms.
15. Unlike men, women DO NOT experience a refractory period.

Why Women Have Sex

"The essence of who we are lies within our ability to express and embrace our unique and individual sexuality. We need to take a more proactive role in managing our sexual health by learning to accept, embody and celebrate our sexual selves and by redefining who we are as sexual beings."

—Dr. TaMara

Psychologists Cindy Meston and David Buss, both professors at the University of Texas at Austin, decided that the topic of why women have sex deserved a book of its own. This book explores the underlying motivations behind women's sexual decisions. The authors conducted extensive research from June 2006 to April 2009. With the collective voices of over 1,000 women from various backgrounds, Meston and Buss identified over 237 different responses. The most frequent reasons were sexual attraction to the person, the desire for physical pleasure, to express affection, to express their love for a person or because they were sexually aroused and wanted release. Other important reasons included retaliation for a mate's indiscretion, bartering for household chores, pleasure seeking, increasing social status, making a mate jealous, boosting confidence, establishing an emotional connection, sense of obligation, for love, punishment, deception, mate security, health benefits, security, sexual economics, evolutionary reasons and so much more. Meston and

Buss also offer interesting insight into female sexuality from an evolutionary and biopsychosocial perspective that is backed by research.

Women's sexuality is more complex than men's. For example, women
are more contextual than men—they are more easily distracted from
sexual cues by what is going on in their environment—and this necessarily means that sexual desire is more multifaceted in women. Also, women
are less connected with their genitals than are men. For example, when
a man has an erection, he generally feels sexually aroused and wants to
have sex. On the contrary, women may experience genital cues, but they
most often go unnoticed and even when they are noticed, women usually
do not respond to the cues because of all the other things she has going
on—both internally and contextually. It's harder for women to tune these
things out and just focus on the physiological genital sensations. In other
words, a woman will usually ignore the cues because she is less driven by
the intrinsic urges. Men, on the other hand, are more likely to respond to
the opportunity and cues. That is not to say that men are so simple that
they have sex simply because they get an intrinsic urge and erection, but
it does mean that women are, quite frankly, more complicated.

While women who answered Meston and Buss's survey presented
some limitations and criticisms and certainly don't represent every
woman, nor will an anonymous online poll tell us everything we need to
know, this study does present a great starting point to begin the discussion into understanding women's sexualities.

Meston and Buss's research also did a number of good things for
women's sexuality. It opened up an otherwise stigmatized and taboo conversation about sexuality, especially in the area of sexual dysfunction. The
research encouraged more open dialogue about women's sexuality and
more women felt comfortable admitting to, and seeking help for, their
sexual concerns. The research also brought attention to the fact that there
are important differences between men and women that need to be stud-
ied if we are to ever find effective treatments for women's sexual concerns.
There is so much left to be learned about women's sexuality nevertheless,
I AM Sex provides an opportunity to embrace what we know so far.

WHY AM I THINKING ABOUT SEX?

Q. *How do you know when you're truly over someone?*

A. *Very good question! You will know that you are truly over someone when: 1) What that person does or says can no longer affect you, one way or the other. You won't feel the need to respond. 2) When you see that person with or without someone, it does not bother you. You can smile, acknowledge them and continue on your way without being devastated. 3) You don't have to go out of your way to avoid them. Changing your routine indicates that there's still some emotional tie that has power of you and 4) When you don't wish any harm or ill-intent on the person and you can genuinely wish them well. This is a sign indicating that you've healed and put closure to that area of your life.*

Pearls of Wisdom: Did you know that the body and brain remembers great sex?? Great sexual experiences gets imprinted into cell memory, making a great lover hard to forget.

SEX ON THE BRAIN

Have you ever wondered why it seems like some people always have sex on the brain? Or perhaps, why men have this uncontrollable urge for sex? Why women feel this undeniable attraction to someone they've had sex with? How does love at first sight become more than fantasy? The answer to why and how are caused by tiny cocktails with incredible potencies. No, they aren't drinks found in any bar or nightclub. These are chemical cocktails called hormones; which are served up by our own bodies. And the mastermind at the helm of these concoctions is our very own brain. Thanks to the mighty brain, certain hormones help to regulate and control our sexual desires, attractions and how we love.

The chemicals and hormones in our brain are working for and against us in the evolutionary design of sex; they keep us wanting it and ultimately coming back for more and more. Why? The desire to produce babies and expand the human race is naturally inherent. But, we have to want and enjoy sex in order to continue our species; therefore, these notorious instigators of our brain are always working and affecting us. Unfortunately, these master manipulators can sometimes temporarily affect our ability to think clearly. For example, the more we do the "horizontal mambo" with someone, the more we become bonded to them. One day, we may wake up and find ourselves in a relationship with someone whom we may not really know. It seems to have been an illusion of what we wanted to see, an unfortunate experience for some of us from the pleasure center players.

Well, who exactly are these "Pleasure Center Players?"

It's important that we become intimately acquainted with these pleasure center players. The more we know about them, the better we will understand our sometimes insatiable appetite for sex, love, attraction and sexual desires. And the more we're able to understand, the better chances we can navigate our own thoughts and behaviors for sex. So, let's begin, shall we?

Player # 1—Dopamine, aka "The Activator"
When we're head over heels in love or having sexual desires, there's an active increase in the areas of our brain associated with romantic feelings triggered by "the activator," dopamine. The activator is the key to activating the pleasure center of our brain. When released, it produces feelings of pleasure and satisfaction when we're doing things that we really enjoy. Dopamine production occurs during the excitement phase of sex and becomes the building block of arousal and desire. At the moment of orgasm, it is fully released followed by an immediate drop in level. Dopamine can also be highly addictive and some scientists have equated it to the brain pattern and rush experienced by heroin or cocaine users. This could explain one of the reasons why orgasm feels so incredible. Orgasms give you the highest dose of natural dopamine. Who needs drugs when you can just have orgasms?

Player # 2—Prolactin, aka The "Ahhh" Moment!
Prolactin is the afterglow chemical that creates the ahhh feeling. . It is responsible for the refractory period that happens after a man

ejaculates or a woman has a clitoral orgasm. Although these periods act differently for everyone, prolactin is the culprit behind it every time. During sexual arousal there is a peak, and then a crash—that tired feeling after sex. This is because the dopamine-prolactin effect causes a spike, followed by an immediate drop. Prolactin also helps to regulate our sex drive. If the brain isn't producing enough of it, there is only the desire to have sex. However if the brain is producing is too much Prolactin, it can repress the libido and result in a loss of sexual arousal completely. In addition, Prolactin is very important during pregnancy. It stimulates the mammary glands to produce milk and assists in the fetal development of the lungs and immune system.

Player # 3—Oxytocin, aka The Bonder

In some cases, prolactin can create a disconnect between partners and cause them to pull away from each other after sex, but thank goodness oxytocin (player # 3) is there to run damage control! Oxytocin, affectionately labeled "the bonding hormone," is another chemical hormone that is released during sexual activity. It produces feelings of trust, emotional intimacy, relaxation, attachment and contentment between people. It calms the spirit and lifts moods, reducing fear and anxiety and allowing a feeling of safety in the arms of your Beloved. One of the best things about oxytocin is that it definitely believes in reciprocity—the more you give, the more you get! Nonsexual touch can also increase levels of oxytocin. Our pleasure center actually becomes more responsive and releases high levels of oxytocin when we touch, nurture and care for others. Just a 20-30 second hug can work wonders for both men and women. Oxytocin also provides balance between the highs of dopamine and lows of prolactin. So, if you are looking to create lasting bonds and to balance the effects of the dopamine and prolactin, then do something sweet for someone you care about by giving them a loving stroke and/or telling them how you feel about them.

Player # 4—Phenylethylamine (PEA), aka The Love Potion
PEA is known as the "love chemical." It's the reason that we all can experience the "in love" tendency. It has us thinking about and wanting to be with our Beloved all of the time. Under the intoxicating influence of PEA, our Beloved can do no wrong. PEA production commonly lasts for about 1 to 24 months. As soon as the production stops, the honeymoon may slow down or come to a screeching halt. The rose-colored glasses come off and things in your partner that never bothered you before suddenly begin to irritate you. The relationship may begin to suffer or eventually end because we are simply not hardwired to maintain that level of PEA production. But, all hope is not lost! The great news is that besides falling in love, PEA production can be simulated by participating in thrill-seeking activities like sky diving and eating of certain foods like chocolate! So even after the effects of PEA have trickled off with the help of oxytocin, thrill seeking or a little chocolate, we can still love and continue to form lasting bonds with our Beloved and to stay connected, falling in love again and again!

Learning to Balance it all...
With all of the ups, downs and hormonal shifts happening during attraction, sexual arousal, ejaculation and orgasm, it is important that we learn how to be aware of them and find balance as we enter into relationships and love play. With awareness and practice, we can participate in activities or do things to produce and/or activate our Pleasure Center Players. Not having any awareness of neurochemistry and how it can wreak havoc on our relationships puts us at a huge disadvantage and increases the chances of relationship failures. When we are aware of these shifts within their entirety, then things can be easily understood within ourselves or a partner who may also be experiencing these hormonal highs and lows. Understanding these things about ourselves and our partners can help both to have patience and compassion with one another. Let a place of balance be a positive arsenal for the journey of love ahead!

Human Sexual Response Cycle

THE SEXUAL RESPONSE CYCLE REFERS to the sequence of physiological changes that occur in the body as a person becomes sexually aroused. Knowing how your body responds during each phase of the cycle can enhance your relationship and help you pinpoint the cause of any potential sexual dysfunction.

During the 1950s and 1960s, William Masters and Virginia Johnson conducted many important studies within the field of human sexuality. In 1966, in their book *Human Sexual Response*, they detailed a four-stage model of physiological changes of humans during sexual stimulation. These phases, in order of their occurrence, are the excitement phase, plateau phase, orgasmic phase and resolution phase. Both men and women experience these phases, although the timing usually is different. For example, it is unlikely that both partners will reach orgasm at the same time. In addition, the intensity of the response and the time spent in each phase varies from person to person. Understanding these differences may help partners better understand one another's bodies and responses, and enhance the sexual experience and increase sexual pleasure.

THE EXCITEMENT PHASE
The excitement phase, also known as the arousal phase, is the first stage of the human sexual response cycle. It occurs as the result of

physical or mental erotic stimuli, such as kissing, petting, or viewing erotic images that lead to sexual arousal. During the excitement stage, the body prepares for sexual intercourse. Heart rate and blood pressure increase, body muscles tense, sexual flush occurs, nipples become erect, genital and pelvic blood vessels become engorged, and involuntary and voluntary muscles contract. The vagina lengthens and widens, the clitoris swells and enlarges, breasts increase in size, the labia swell and separate, the vagina becomes lubricated, and the uterus rises slightly. Vaginal lubrication is the key indicator of sexual excitement. The excitement phase can last from several minutes to several hours.

THE PLATEAU PHASE

The plateau phase is the highest moment of sexual excitement before orgasm, may be achieved, lost, and regained several times without the occurrence of orgasm. Breathing rate, heart rate, and blood pressure further increase, sexual flush deepens, and muscle tension increases. There is a sense of impending orgasm. The clitoris becomes extremely sensitive and withdraws slightly beneath the clitoral hood, the Bartholin's glands[1] lubricate, the areolae around the nipples become larger, the labia continue to swell, the uterus tips to stand high in the abdomen, and the "orgasmic platform" develops (the lower vagina swells, narrows, and tightens).

During the plateau stage, there is a sense of impending orgasm. Prolonged time in the plateau phase without progression to the orgasmic phase may result in frustration if continued for too long. For those who never achieve orgasm, this is the peak of sexual excitement.

ORGASM PHASE

Orgasm is the conclusion of the plateau phase. At the moment of orgasm, the sexual tension that has been building throughout the

---

1 More about what Bartholin's glands are later.

body is released, and the body releases chemicals called endorphins, which cause a sense of well-being. Orgasms in females can vary widely from woman to woman, but in general, they are accompanied by quick cycles of muscle contraction in the lower pelvic muscles which surround both the anus and the primary sexual organs. Orgasms are often associated with other involuntary actions, including vocalizations and muscular spasms in other areas of the body.

RESOLUTION PHASE

The resolution phase occurs after orgasm and allows the muscles to relax, blood pressure to drop and the body to slow down from its excited state. The refractory period, which is part of the resolution phase, is the time frame in which usually a man is unable to orgasm again. Though women can also experience a very brief refractory period, they can either enter the resolution stage or return to the excitement or plateau stage immediately following orgasm. After the initial orgasm, subsequent orgasms for women may also be stronger or more pleasurable as the stimulation accumulates. According to Masters and Johnson, women have the ability to orgasm again very quickly, as long as they have effective stimulation. They are, as a result, able to have multiple orgasms in a relatively short period of time. For some women, the clitoris is very sensitive after climax, making additional stimulation initially painful. In this case, it may be best to just cuddle after an orgasm until the hypersensitivity of the clitoris has subsided.

Although Masters and Johnson's model of human sexual response has been widely accepted as a valid and credible model of human sexuality, there has been some criticism of the model. Some of the criticisms of the model include:

* Defining sexual response exclusively as a physiological/biological response

* The lack of acknowledgement of the emotional, mental, spiritual, social, cultural, etc. impact on sexual response, arousal and desire
* The lack of unison between emotional, mental and genital arousal
* Failure to account for differences between men and women's varying response to sexual stimuli, thus pathologizing natural female responses
* Failure to acknowledge that some women will not move progressively and sequentially through the linear order
* Assumptions that female sexual response is largely a reaction and response to and dependent on their partner
* Failure to acknowledge desire as a key initiator in sexual activity
* The lack of acknowledging pleasure and satisfaction as key to sexual response

Additionally, researchers Helen Singer Kaplan, Rosemary Basson, Beverly Whipple and Karen Brash-McGreer argue that this model does not accurately explain the complexities of the female sexual response cycle.

In 1979, Helen Singer Kaplan introduced a modified, tri-phasic model of sexual response which includes an interconnected cycle of desire, excitement, and orgasm. The unique aspect of Kaplan's model is that it considered desire as a precursor to excitement, which had largely been ignored in Masters and Johnson's sexual response cycle. Although Kaplan's model now included desire into the equation, it was still a linear model that still focused on orgasm as the end result of sexual satisfaction. Additionally, Kaplan's model of sexual response still did not account for the differences between men and women and the variation of "normal" response to sexual stimuli. It also did not determine if sexual desire was completely necessary for sexual arousal. Critics of this model believe that it is still a better indicator of the male sexual response cycle.

In 1997, well-known sexologist Beverly Whipple and her partner, Karen Brash-McGreer, offered the first non-linear approach to female sexual response. This model acknowledged that sexual pleasure and satisfaction was an essential motivating factor in a woman's desire to engage in sexual activity. Whipple and Brash-McGreer's model is based on four stages that somewhat parallel the linear model of sexual response. The four stages include: seduction (encompassing desire), sensations (excitement and plateau), surrender (orgasm), and reflection (resolution). Whipple and Brash-McGreer asserted that if a woman did not receive pleasure and satisfaction during a sexual experience, that she would be less likely to desire to repeat the sexual experience.

Rosemary Basson's model of sexual response also took a circular approach. In 2000, Bassoon proposed a model based on both biological and psychological response. She believed that sexual drive is shaped by sexual stimuli, sexual arousal, desire, emotional and physical satisfaction and emotional intimacy. The thought behind the circular model is that once a woman is sexually aroused, she becomes motivated to flow continuously into each phase, becoming sexually fulfilled. The Basson model clarifies that the goal of sexual activity for women is not necessarily orgasm, but rather personal satisfaction, which can manifest as physical satisfaction (orgasm) and/or emotional satisfaction (a feeling of intimacy and connection with a partner).[2] Basson's model also accounts for sexual satisfaction in long-term relationships in which relationship satisfaction, intimacy and emotional closeness with one's Beloved may predispose a woman to participate in sexual play.

There has also been criticism of Kaplan's; Whipple and Brash-McGreer's; and Basson's models. Nevertheless, these models provide significant insight into women's sexual response. However, more research needs to be done in this area to show whether the circular model more accurately describes women's sexual response.

---

2 Basson, R. "Female Sexual Response: The Role of Drugs in the Management of Sexual Dysfunction. "*Obstet Gynecol* 2001;98:350-353.

DR. TAMARA'S PROPOSED MODEL OF FEMALE SEXUAL RESPONSE

I have a deep appreciation and respect for all of the conceptual models of human sexual response. I use Basson's in my practice to help my clients understand how sex really works for us. I also use Masters and Johnson's model because it offers a foundation for how we understand sexual response. Although I have an appreciation and respect for all the aforementioned models of sexual response, I, too, find them to be limited in that they do not take into account all the various influences on sexual response.

My model conceptualizes and acknowledges that female sexual functioning proceeds in a more complex and circuitous manner than male sexual functioning and that female functioning is dramatically and significantly affected by numerous physiological and psychosocial issues, being heavily embedded in relationship issues, in culture and ethnicity, religion, body image, education, sexual education, self-confidence, and many other things—satisfaction with the relationship, self-image, previous negative sexual experiences, etc.

Sexual response is traditionally only described in terms of physical events (heart rate, blood pressure, engorgement, etc...). While sexual response may be observed in the body, it is experienced cognitively and psychologically, and our subjective experience of sexual response should be included in descriptions.

I offer a model of sexual responses that is based on what I call the "Dimensions of Sexuality." My proposed model is more like a bicycle wheel, with the inner and outer wheel being connected by spokes. The inner wheel is who we are, the outer wheel is our sexual response. The spokes of the wheel are the various social determinants, environmental factors, life stressors, relational factors, intergenerational patterns, genetics, etc. that all impact our sexual response in the Dimensions of Sexuality: emotional, mental, spiritual, social, legal, economical, chemical, energetical, institutional, political and physical. The inner self, outer self, Dimensions of Sexuality and sexual response are all intertwined to create a set of complex, divergent responses. Sexuality and our response to it is not linear or circular; it's truly a beautiful, fluid response based on any given external or internal stimuli.

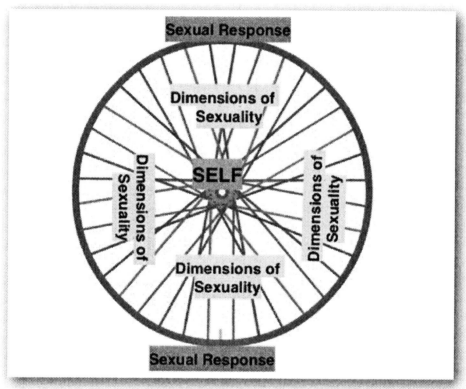

Figure 1.Dr. TaMara's Model of Sexual Response

THE IMPORTANCE OF UNDERSTANDING THE MODELS

Learning about different sexual models can be tremendously relieving to both parties. Women can understand that they are not abnormal because they don't think about sex as often as their partner does, or feel aroused spontaneously, as he sometimes does. Men can be reassured that simply because she does not experience desire in the same pattern as he does, this does not mean she is not attracted to him or unable to be aroused.

Sharing this information is helpful in providing a basic understanding of sexual response. It is not meant to categorize sexual response into a box. Many people will read about human sexual response and consider it to be what's "healthy" or "normal."

As you can see, the variety of sexual response models demonstrate that sex is complex. There is no way to truly measure sexual response. In reality, the sexual response is an imposition on a very fluid process of excitement, arousal, tension, release, and more. At times there may be a "typical" pattern, but other times, things will be completely different. Our sexual response flows and changes, and often the descriptions you hear won't exactly match your experience. This doesn't mean there's anything wrong with you; it is just an example of how sexual response is truly unique to each of us.

Two key insights: one, female sexual desire is generally more responsive than spontaneous. That is, we are more likely to respond to sexual stimuli—thoughts, sights, smells, and sounds—than we are to spark an interest in sex out of thin air. Two, emotional intimacy matters to women. That doesn't sound like a news flash, but in the realm of the biological sciences, it's news—trust me!

Finally, it is important to note that there is a difference between arousal and desire. Arousal, which causes lubrication, is physiological, and the desire to have sex is psychological. Essentially, a woman can have the desire to have sex but not be aroused, which means that there may be some type of issue going on that needs to be addressed. So in other words, she could want to have sex but her body may not get aroused, and vice versa.

BENEFITS OF THE HUMAN SEXUAL RESPONSE MODELS

There are numerous benefits of understanding the human sexual response model which include:

* Understanding the physiological response to sexual arousal
* Identification of sexual triggers
* Helping to increase sexual pleasure
* Exploring and understanding past sexual experiences.

Female Reproductive System

THE FEMALE REPRODUCTIVE SYSTEM IS actually pretty amazing. It is a collection of organs that work together for the purpose of producing a new life and experiencing sexual pleasure. The reproductive system is among the most important systems in the entire body. Without the ability to experience sexual pleasure and reproduce, the human race would surely die off.

Reproductive health is influenced by many factors. These include age, lifestyle, habits, genetics, use of medicines and exposure to chemicals in the environment. These influences may cause a woman to experience reproductive health challenges and quality of life issues such as infertility or sexual dysfunctions.

Reproductive health problems can also be harmful to overall health and impair a person's ability to enjoy a sexual relationship. Many problems of the reproductive system can be corrected with proper treatment from a multidisciplinary team of care providers such as gynecologists, obstetricians, sexologists and sex therapists.

Mound of Venus

Carefully created to provide you pleasure
cultivating like a gardener I prune
shaving and trimming to perfection so smooth
you touch my mound of Venus
captivated by her beauty

suspended from her aura so breathtaking
you long to feel her so deep inside
you must,
experience her so surreal
into the Heavens……..yes, she is miraculous
the power to give life
how extraordinaire
her pheromones drive you wild
in confidence she controls all
to her feminine wiles you so willingly submit
my mound of Venus
to it, be the glory!

The female reproductive system includes the external genitalia and internal organs which work closely together to help the system function properly and provide pleasure. The more that is known about the reproductive system and how it functions, the better one is able to provide personal pleasure. Let's begin this fantastic journey into the female reproductive system!

First up is the clitoris…one of the most infamous, misunderstood and under appreciated organs. According to some researchers, stimulation of this organ accounts for 50 to 75 percent of most orgasms. Over 90 percent of women experience their first orgasm through its direct stimulation. Even more amazingly, most women experience multiple orgasms as a result of direct or indirect stimulation of this special spot of precious pleasure. With over 8,000 nerve endings—twice as many as the "mighty" male penis, it's no wonder why women can achieve multiple, mind-blowing orgasms.

So what exactly is she—the clitoris? Many women complain that their partner can't find her, mistreat her, or don't spend nearly enough time getting to know her. And the vast majority of women do stimulate her in order to enhance their sexual experience! She is a key player to sexual pleasure. She's a small, round blossom of pinkish or brownish flesh located just above the vaginal opening. A true cutie, but shy at times! She's usually hiding under her custom designed house, a soft fold of tissue called the "clitoral hood" that helps to protect it from over stimulation. Her size and shape will differ from woman to woman, but on average she's about two and a half to four inches long, similar to the length of a flaccid penis. However, it's important to note that her size does not correlate with the amount of pleasure she gives. Treat her right—with the right stimulation, results of magnificent multitude can be achieved, no matter her length!

There's more to her than meets the eye! Only a small portion of her can be seen by the naked eye, since about 75 percent of her is hidden internally. Most people only focus on her pretty bold head or "glans". But, the clitoris is actually a complex network of nerves that stretch throughout the vagina and up into her woman's body. Some of her hidden internal parts include erectile tissue, glands, muscles, blood vessels, and nerves. Internally, the clitoris has a bulb winged-like figure that is reminiscent of a wishbone and sits on both sides of the urethra. These pretty wings are made of erectile tissue that extend beneath the inner lips of the vagina, and they fill with blood when her woman is aroused!

Once aroused, her bulb fills with blood, increasing her size and sensitivity, which may retract her hood to reveal her head. At the peak of pleasure or orgasm, she will return to her petite size. But, sometimes when orgasm isn't achieved or for some other reason her bulb may remain full. If it's for longer than a few hours, her condition and discomfort is pretty much the male equivalent of "blue balls."

In truth, every woman is very unique, and so is her clitoris. Not only in appearance, but in the way to engage it and maintain a satisfying level of sexual arousal as well. The sensitivity of the clitoris and how she likes it to be handled for pleasure varies greatly from woman to woman. The direct approach is not always the best approach when it comes to the clitoris. Some women do not enjoy direct stimulation because the overall feeling can be very intense which may eventually cause pain for them. Other women enjoy the intensity and direct pressure and/or stimulation of their clitoris because it feels exhilarating for them. Then there are others who prefer stimulation from the side area or on top of the clitoral hood and the feeling is just as breathtaking If you or your partner is uncertain of your level of clitoral sensitivity, it's always best to start out gently, nice and slow, then vary your touch depending on the reaction being conveyed.

Can we all just face the clitoral truth? The clitoris, with its miraculous and mysterious power demands respect, appreciation and attention. The more we understand the center of a woman's pleasure, the more we're able to facilitate experiences of unparalleled bliss.

Next up is the vulva, which is home to the clitoris. The vulva is the collective name for the external female genitalia located in the pubic region of the body. The vulva surrounds the external ends of the urethral opening and the vagina. In addition to the clitoris, the vulva includes labia majora, labia minora and Bartholin's gland.

Affectionately referred to as "the lips," and literally translating as "large lips," the labia majora enclose and protect the other external reproductive organs. The labia majora are relatively large and fleshy, and are comparable to the scrotum in males. The labia majora contain sweat and oil-secreting glands. After puberty, the labia majora are covered with hair.

Just inside the labia majora, and surround the openings to the vagina and urethra lies the delicate folds of the labia minora. Literally translated as "small lips," the labia minora can be very small or up to two inches wide.

Located slightly behind and to the left and right of the opening of the vagina are the Bartholin glands. These two pea sized glands secrete mucus to provide lubrication to the vagina when a woman is sexually aroused. The fluid helps slightly moisten the labial opening of the vagina, to help make contact with this highly sensitive area more arousing and comfortable for the woman.

The internal reproductive organs in the female include: ovaries, fallopian tubes, uterus, cervix and vagina.

The ovaries are a pair of small glands about the size and shape of almonds, located on the left and right sides of the pelvic body cavity lateral to the superior portion of the uterus. Ovaries produce female sex hormones such as estrogen and progesterone as well as ova (commonly called "eggs"), the female gametes. Ova are produced from oocyte cells that slowly develop throughout a woman's early life and reach maturity after puberty. Each month during ovulation, a mature ovum is released. The ovum travels from the ovary to the fallopian tube, where it may be fertilized before reaching the uterus.

Pearls of Wisdom:
During fetal life, there are about 6 million to 7 million eggs. From this time, no new eggs are produced. At birth, there are approximately 1 million eggs; and by the time of puberty, only about 300,000 remain. Of these, only 300 to 400 will mature to ovulation during a woman's reproductive lifetime. Fertility can drop as a woman ages due to decreasing number and quality of the remaining eggs.

The fallopian tubes are a pair of muscular tubes that are attached to left and right top corners of the uterus and extend to the edge of the ovaries. The fallopian tubes end in a funnel-shaped structure called the infundibulum, which is covered with small finger-like projections called fimbriae. The fimbriae swipe over the outside of the ovaries to pick up released ova and carry them into the infundibulum for transport to the uterus. The inside of each fallopian tube is covered in cilia that work with the smooth muscle of the tube to carry the ovum to the uterus. Conception, the fertilization of an egg by a sperm, normally occurs in the fallopian tubes. The fertilized egg then moves to the uterus, where it implants into the lining of the uterine wall.

The uterus, also known as the womb, is a hollow, muscular, pear-shaped organ located behind and above the urinary bladder. It is connected to the two fallopian tubes on its top end and to the vagina (via the cervix) on its bottom end. The main function of the uterus is to support the developing fetus during pregnancy. The inner lining of the uterus, known as the endometrium, provides support to the embryo during early development. The visceral muscles of the uterus contract during childbirth to push the fetus through the cervix and the vagina.

The cervix is a cylinder-shaped neck of tissue that connects the vagina and uterus. The cervix is made of cartilage covered by smooth, moist tissue, and is about one inch across. Its name, cervix, comes from the Latin word meaning "neck" due to its role as the narrow connection between the larger body of the uterus above, and the vagina below.

The cervix can be broken down into several anatomically distinct regions:

* The cervical canal is the hollow orifice through the cervix that connects the uterine cavity to the hollow lumen of the vagina.
* Connecting the cervical canal to the lumen of the vagina is a small circular opening surrounded by the external tissue of the cervix also known as the external os.
* Connecting the cervical canal to the uterine cavity is a small circular opening where the cervical canal narrows before opening into the uterus, also known as the internal os.

The cervix produces cervical mucus that changes in consistency during the menstrual cycle to prevent or promote pregnancy. Lining the inside of the cervix is a thin layer of endometrium containing the epithelial cells that constantly produce cervical mucus. The cervical mucus fills the cervical canal and forms a mucus plug, blocking the flow of material between the uterus and the vagina. Around the time of ovulation, the consistency of the cervical mucus becomes much thinner, allowing the passage of sperm into the uterus for fertilization. The cervix plays vital roles in the control of movement into and out of the uterus, protection of the fetus during pregnancy, and the delivery of the fetus during childbirth. Additionally, during pregnancy the cervix and its mucus plug protect the developing fetus by sealing the uterus from possible contamination by external pathogens. During menstruation, the smooth muscle tissue in the myometrium of the cervix dilates to allow the passage of menstrual flow and may cause sensations of pain and discomfort known as menstrual cramps. Additionally, during sexual intercourse, the cervical mucus helps sperm move from the vagina through the cervix into the uterus.

Last, but certainly not the least of the internal organs of the female reproductive system is the vagina. The vagina is an elastic, muscular tube that connects the cervix of the uterus to the exterior of the body. It is located inferior to the uterus and posterior to the urinary bladder. The vagina functions as the receptacle for the penis during sexual intercourse and carries sperm to the uterus and fallopian tubes. It also serves as the birth canal by stretching to allow delivery of the fetus during childbirth. During menstruation, the menstrual flow exits the body via the vagina.

Q. *I was talking with a group of girlfriends and one of them mentioned that she thought about trying g-spot injections to enhance her orgasms. I've never heard of this before. What are g-spot injections? Does it work and what are your thoughts on this?*

A. *G-Spot injection, also known as G-Spot Amplification, is a procedure that can temporarily enlarge the G-Spot and enhance sexual sensitivity and pleasure during intercourse. The procedure takes about 10-15 minutes and is usually performed in a doctor's office. During the procedure, a small amount of collagen is directly placed into the G-Spot, increasing it to about the size of a quarter. Each shot lasts about 4 months and the results vary from woman to woman. Repeat injections are required to maintain the effect. There is a laundry list of potential risks associated with this procedure. My concern with the G-Spot Amplification is that there has not been a documented study on the safety and efficacy of the procedure. It is an invasive procedure that involves inserting something into the vagina that has never been approved by the FDA (Food and Drug Administration). Another concern is that over time the procedure can cause permanent scarring to the G-Spot erectile tissue which can lead to female erectile dysfunction and other sexual dysfunctions. If your concern is the inability to experience orgasm or if the desire is to enhance your sexual life, then you may want to consider working with a sex counselor or therapist to address your concern in a more holistic way. Medical intervention is not always the best method. We're always looking for quick fixes for lots of things in our lives, and sexuality is no different. However, it's going to take more than a shot to create an orgasmic sex life!*

What would a conversation about the vagina be without a mention of the G-Spot? There are very few issues in sexology, sexual medicine and sex therapy that instigate so much interest, debate and controversy among clinicians and practitioners than the G-spot. One of the main reasons why the G-spot seems to garner much preoccupation and seems to be quite mysterious is because it seems as if not everybody can find it, nor is every woman able to orgasm through it.

The 17th-century Dutch physician Regnier de Graaf described female ejaculation and referred to an erogenous zone in the vagina that he linked with the male prostate; this zone was later reported by the German gynecologist Ernst Gräfenberg in the fifties. Beverly Whipple, a certified sex educator and counselor, and John D. Perry, an ordained minister, psychologist, and sexologist, named the G-spot after Ernst Grafenberg. Dr. Grafenberg was the first modern physician to describe the area and argue for its importance in female sexual pleasure.

The "Grafenberg Spot," or what is more popularly known as the G-spot, is a spongy tissue that is located on the vagina's inner wall. When stimulated, this area of the vagina can lead to strong sexual arousal, powerful orgasms and female ejaculation. This bean-shaped spot is located one to three inches up the anterior vaginal wall. It has also been reported that this highly sensitive area may be part of the female prostate.

FINDING THE G SPOT

The G-spot is just one of many glands that are positioned on a woman's vaginal wall. Every woman has a G-spot in her body. The female G-spot has a similar structure and functions much like a man's prostate. As a matter of fact, the male prostate is frequently referred to as a male G-spot since the stimulation of the prostate can result in great sexual pleasure. G-spot stimulation and orgasm has also been known to result in the phenomenon known as female ejaculation.

The key factor in finding the G-spot is becoming intimately acquainted with one's body. There are several ways individuals can try to stimulate the G-spot. Because the G-spot is embedded in the muscle of the vaginal wall, it may be difficult to initially find it. It may require a little patience and effort. Every woman will respond differently; however, the more aroused the woman is, the larger and more sensitive the G-spot becomes, making it easier to find. The initial stimulation may cause a woman to feel a strong urge to urinate. However, this sensation passes after a short while and will be replaced by feelings of pleasure and arousal.

Using a G-spot vibrator may be useful in locating the G-spot. This sex toy is specifically designed to help stimulate the G-spot. There are a wide variety to choose from, depending on your mood for exploration and creativity! These vibrators come in a variety of colors, materials and prices. Some are actually waterproof! You can purchase one of these fun toys from any adult toy retailer.

Although all females have a G-spot, it is estimated that only10-20% of females are able to experience ejaculation. Responses vary, ranging from a very light sprinkle up to a great gush of large quantities of fluid. The elusive female ejaculation commonly known as gushing or squirting is a phenomenon that has been glamorized by the adult entertainment industry, but is actually more real than you think; that is, of course, minus the lights, camera, props and the beauty of editing! According to research conducted by Dr. Beverly Whipple, one of the world's leading pioneers on the G-spot and the science of orgasm, many women admit to experiencing female ejaculation during sex—solo or with a partner.

What is female ejaculation? Female ejaculation refers to a watery fluid that originates in the G-Spot and is secreted by the Skenes/Paraurethral glands through the urethra before and/or during orgasm. Although the fluid released during female ejaculation comes from the urethra, rest assured it is not urine. The fluid is female ejaculate, and it comes from the ducts around the urethra, not from the bladder, where urine is stored. The reason why people may confuse female ejaculate with urine is due to the fact that female ejaculate can also sometimes travel back up into the bladder, which is called retrograde ejaculation. Because the female ejaculate may mix with urine and even share some of the same properties of urine-urea and creatinine—many people think that it is urine; however, that is not the case.

Female ejaculate is also distinctly different from normal vaginal fluid. Normal vaginal fluid can vary in taste, smell, color and consistency depending on the menstrual cycle, hormonal levels, food intake, presence of infection etc. Female ejaculate, on the other hand is fairly consistent in the taste, smell, color and consistency. It is a sweet smelling, watery type of fluid and is not the typical fluid that one sees when a woman is wet from sexual arousal or having had an orgasm.

So what causes female ejaculation? During sexual arousal, the G-Spot becomes enlarged and the tissue surrounding the urethra becomes engorged with blood and the Skenes/Paraurethral glands begin to produce and fill with fluid. The rhythmic pressure from fingers, toys, a penis, or the contractions of orgasm pushes the fluid out through the urethral opening, causing ejaculation. The amount of fluid expelled during ejaculation can vary from woman to woman; while the average amount is somewhere around two tablespoons, this can be affected by how hydrated a woman is and how much she pushes while ejaculating.

Can every women experience female ejaculation? All women have the Paraurethral/Skenes glands, so all women are capable of producing this fluid and can eventually achieve female ejaculation! Interestingly enough, many women experience ejaculation during sex, but do not realize what's happening and as a result, they cut the experience short for fear of "urinating on their partner." That fear leads to clenching down of the pubococcygeus (PC) muscles, which stops the fluid from coming out. The inability to relax, bear down and push prevents the release of the ejaculate. This inability usually comes down to a matter of inhibitions regarding sexuality, embarrassment, guilt, unfamiliarity of female reproductive system, not being in touch with one's own body, not having a thorough understanding of female ejaculation, lack of connection and/or sexual compatibility with partner, and stress.

How can a woman increase her chances of experiencing female ejaculation? The first step is to STOP TRYING! Like exploring everything else new in your experience of sex, you should work towards it, but not put unnecessary stresses on yourself or your partner by making it your goal. Having goal-oriented sex almost always ensures that you will not reach your sexual goal. Addressing any psychological barriers that may contribute to an inability to fulfill sexual desires may also be helpful and/or it may be just be a matter of finding the right technique.

The most simple and effective way to bring yourself or your partner one step closer to allowing the waters to flow from within is by including some of the following tips into your regular sex play:

* Strengthen your PC Muscles. Being able to contract and release your PC muscle can help with achieving female ejaculation.
* Add clitoral stimulation to your G-spot stimulation. Multiple forms of stimulation help to increase levels of arousal.
* Locate your G-Spot. Try using a G-spot stimulator to help locate your G-Spot. The G-Spot is usually much easier to locate after the first orgasm.
* Try to urinate before sex play. Emptying your bladder will help to reduce anxiety around urinating on your partner.
* Bear down and push when you feel like you are about to have an orgasm, rather than clenching tight. This will help to force out

any fluid that has built up in the Skenes/Paraurethral glands. Whatever you do, don't stop pushing—just allow the fluid to flow. The orgasm will be very intense and pleasurable.

❋ Seek the advice of a professional sex coach, therapist or counselor. There may be some deeper issue blocking your ability to experience your sexual desires.

Introducing something new in your sex play for the first time can seem embarrassing, or even a little scary. Try to make yourself as comfortable as possible and try to enjoy what the experience has to offer. Create a space for yourself that will let you and/or your partner explore your body in without judgment, barriers and goals. Give yourself the permission and freedom to let yourself go…then do it! But most importantly, have fun! Remember, the journey is just as important as the destination!

Q. *I listened to most of the squirting episode on your radio show; however; I did not hear an answer to the question on how you prepare a man for squirting. I have been a squirter for quite a few years now (I thought I had a gift…lol), even before I ever heard of anyone else doing it. I do not squirt across the room; I just "flood" (for a lack of a better word) the bed. My boyfriend gets freaked out from it which makes me tense up and not able to have an orgasm at all. I'm literally starting to suppress my orgasms because now I'm afraid that I might squirt and he will literally stop right in the middle of having sex. I've shown him that the fluid is not pee, but he still thinks it is. In addition, he will not give me oral sex because he fears that I might come all over him. I love the messiness of sex; however; I can't enjoy our sex as much because I can't control the size of my orgasms!!! I love him and want to stay with him, but this is making it hard for me to stay faithful. What is your advice? HELP!!!*

A. *You are blessed with a gift of being in touch with your sexuality. You are able to freely submit yourself to the beauty of female ejaculation, something that so many women desire to experience, but for many reasons do not. Unfortunately, due to a lack of sexual education among other things,* many people, both men and women, do not understand the phenomenon of female ejaculation. Female ejaculation, also referred to as squirting or gushing, is a natural occurrence resulting from intense G-spot stimulation. It occurs more frequently than one might expect but because some women are not as intimately acquainted with their bodies they are not attune to the experience.

From what I've read, you have already done a fantastic job trying to address your boyfriend's concerns. A couple things come to mind regarding your situation. It seems as though his reservations stem from a fear and/or lack of understanding about female orgasms. It also seems that he may have some inhibitions/hang-ups when it comes to sexual experiences.

As you are already aware, this could become a much bigger issue in your relationship if you both do not address it. I encourage you to continue talking with him prior to the act of sex. Using shows like my radio show and reading books together are great ways to start the conversation. During the conversation, you want to find out the answers to the following questions:

1. What are his fears when it comes to female ejaculation?
2. What is the worst thing that could happen when you ejaculate?
3. What causes him to stop during the middle of sex?
4. What goes through his mind as you are ejaculating?

Finding out the answers to the questions is a good starting point for identifying ways to address his specific concerns.

Suppressing your sexuality is not fair to you! You should be able to explore and share all facets of your sexuality with your partner. Continuing to suppress your sexuality will only result in disappoint, resentment, frustration and as you mentioned, "make it hard to stay faithful." Consider sharing how important it is for you to be able to experience and share your sexuality with him. Also, try explaining to him that your sexual responses are the result of the closeness and intimate bond that the two of you share. Be patient and allow his to ask any questions and share his feelings.

Sexual incompatibility between partners can definitely cause challenges in a relationship. It is important to address them as soon as they come up. Dealing with such issues takes a team approach and willingness to resolve. I encourage you to work together to come up with a sexual script that includes both of your sexual wants, needs and desires so that when played out, you both end up happy and satisfied.

Becoming Intimately Acquainted With Yourself

FOR MANY OF PEOPLE, MASTURBATION or self-pleasure is a taboo topic. There are many harmful myths that exist about masturbation that may cause people to feel uncomfortable. Society and the media do a great job at contributing to the taboo, stigma and negative messages around sexuality. Marketing and advertising companies teach us that our bodies are dirty and disgusting. Constantly being inundated with such messages, beliefs, attitudes and feelings like these contribute to the unhealthy behaviors that put women at risk for HIV and other sexually transmitted infections, victimization, abuse, body image issues, unhealthy relationships, mental health challenges and so much more.

In some cultures and religions, masturbation is considered sinful. This can lead to guilt or shame about the behavior. Negative messages and feelings about masturbation can threaten our health and well-being. People who receive negative messages about masturbation when they are young often carry feelings of shame surrounding sexuality into adulthood which can ultimately affect the way we interact in relationships and experience sexual pleasure.

In order to fully experience your sexuality, you have to move past the shame and peel back the negative and unhealthy layers of intergenerational patterns that surround sexuality. While masturbation was once thought of as a perversion and a sign of a mental problem, masturbation now is regarded as a natural, healthy sexual activity that is pleasurable and safe. According to various studies, masturbation is a very common behavior, even among people who have a sex partner. According to one national study, 95% of males and 89% of females reported that they have masturbated and here are some reasons why.

THE CLITORIS CONNECTION!

Women have been perfectly designed with their own special pleasure spot! Did you know this spot is the only organ in the human body with the sole function of providing pleasure? In fact, most women usually experience their first clitoral orgasm through masturbation. When you know what you need to bring yourself pleasure and orgasm, you strengthen your connection to your body, in addition to experiencing many other health benefits of masturbation.

YOU LEARN MORE ABOUT YOUR BODY

In order to experience pleasure, you have to be intimately acquainted with your body. Understanding your sexual response cycle and how your body changes during each cycle is the hallmark of sexual pleasure. Masturbation is a great way to learn all about your body, your sexual response and sexual triggers. Learning about what feels good to you can increase your chance of experiencing sexual pleasure with sex partners because it enables you to communicate your sexual turn-ons to your partners.

CREATE AN INTIMATE BOND

Some partners use mutual masturbation to discover techniques for a more satisfying sexual and intimate relationship. Through mutual masturbation, you learn about body mapping. This technique helps you learn what spots, various strokes and techniques to use to please your partner and vice versa. In addition, mutual masturbation is a safer way to explore sexual activity with another person because it lowers your risk for unintended pregnancies, HIV and other sexually transmitted infections.

INCREASED CONFIDENCE

There is a correlation between sexuality and confidence. Knowing how your body works and what you're capable of helps to increase your confidence. The more confident you are, the more likely you are able to make better decisions, creating stronger boundaries and facilitate healthier relationships. When you can bring yourself physical pleasure, you don't need someone else to validate you. This, unsurprisingly, leads to higher confidence and increased level of self-care that transcends beyond the bedroom.

Added Health Benefits:
Masturbation provides many health benefits that can help to enhance our physical, emotional, mental, and sexual health. Some of the benefits include:

* Creating a sense of well-being
* Enhancing partnered sexual experiences
* Increasing the ability to have orgasms
* Improving relationship and sexual satisfaction
* Improving sleep
* Increasing confidence self-esteem and improve body image
* Providing sexual pleasure for people without partners
* Providing treatment for some sexual dysfunctions
* Reducing stress
* Relieving sexual tension
* Relieving menstrual cramps
* Strengthening muscle tone in the pelvic and anal areas

Pleasuring oneself is one of the most powerful sexual experiences. The freedom to give yourself the permission to explore your body, the time and space to feel pleasure, and to know that you are worth giving and receiving pleasure are some of the most powerful steps to becoming sexually empowered and liberated! Finally, in the words of Ru Paul, "if you can't love yourself, how in the hell are you going to love someone else?" And if you do decide to show yourself a little love—trust me, you won't go blind!

At the end of the day, only you can decide what is healthy and right for you. If you feel ashamed or guilty about masturbating, consider talking with a sex therapist, educator, counselor, and/or clergy member to explore your beliefs and attitudes regarding sexuality.

PLEASURE EXERCISE

Prepare yourself for pleasure by setting the mood. Seduction is the key! Don't just take off your clothes and get right into it—relax and take your time. Entice yourself by performing a hot and sexy strip tease. Start by turning on your favorite song to get you into the mood. Slowly begin peeling away all your clothes, layer by layer, until you are completely exposed.

Take a relaxing bubble bath. Totally submerge your body in the hot and steamy water. Take deep breaths—inhale through the nose and exhale through the mouth. Massage your entire body as you lather with bubble bath or bath oil. Shave or trim up your private area. After about 30 minutes, dry off your entire body with a warm fluffy towel. Oil your entire body with your favorite body oil. Take your time to massage the oil into your skin.

Use a mirror to explore your lady parts! Use a mirror to explore the outside of your anatomy. Familiarize yourself with all you behold. Admire and appreciate yourself just as you are. As you become more aware of yourself, you will be able to experience more pleasure.

Slowly begin to pleasure yourself by tracing all of your curves and paying special attention to your sweetness. Gently caress your sweet spot using various strokes, motions, speed and pressure to enhance stimulation. Pay close attention to varying sensation as this will help you to be more in tune with your body as well as identify what turns you on. You may also consider using a vibrator to intensify the experience. Lubricant may also provide extra stimulation.

If you really want to heighten your experience, try completing these steps in front of a full-length mirror. If you want to intensify your orgasm, pleasure yourself almost to the point of no return and just before you climax, stop. Do this a few times and this will help to increase your orgasmic intensity.

Pearls of Wisdom: No two vulvas are alike! Just as women are created differently, so are vulvas. Each has its own distinct look. Lips vary in thickness, color, length, and shape. Just like anything else new, this may be weird or uncomfortable at first, but I encourage you to push through the feeling. If uncomfortable, repeat this exercise until you become more comfortable and intimately acquainted with yourself.

The Menstrual Cycle, Pregnancy and Menopause

Q. *Right before my period, I get really horny and I want to have sex all the time. Is this normal?*

A. *Yes, it is natural for women to get "really horny" right before her monthly cycle. You can thank the high levels of estrogen and testosterone that spikes before and during ovulation. That combined with lots of slippery cervical fluids helps to skyrocket your sex drive, which keeps you wanting it more and more!*

Q. *I have noticed changes in my vaginal lubrication. Is this normal?*

A. *The amount consistency, texture, taste, color, and odor can change depending on sexual arousal, the phase of the menstrual cycle, the presence of an infection, certain, genetic factors, and diet. It is important to become intimately acquainted with your vagina's normal lubrication, so if there is a noticeable change in color (i.e. greenish yellow, grayish), consistency (i.e. clumpy white, too runny) and smell (fishy, foul) you can contact your physician to check for a presence of infection.*

The female reproductive cycle is the process of producing an ovum and readying the uterus to receive a fertilized ovum to begin pregnancy. If an ovum is produced but not fertilized and implanted in the uterine wall, the reproductive cycle resets itself through menstruation. The entire reproductive cycle takes about 28 days on average, but may be as short as 24 days or as long as 36 days for some women.

Oogenesis and Ovulation
Under the influence of follicle stimulating hormone (FSH), and luteinizing hormone (LH), the ovaries produce a mature ovum in a process known as ovulation. By about 14 days into the reproductive cycle, an oocyte reaches maturity and is released as an ovum. Although the ovaries begin to mature many oocytes each month, usually only one ovum per cycle is released.

Fertilization
Once the mature ovum is released from the ovary, the fimbriae catch the egg and direct it down the fallopian tube to the uterus. It takes about a week for the ovum to travel to the uterus. If sperm are able to reach and penetrate the ovum, the ovum becomes a fertilized zygote containing a full complement of DNA. After a two-week period of rapid cell division known as the germinal period of development, the zygote forms an embryo. The embryo will then implant itself into the uterine wall and develop there during pregnancy.

Menstruation
While the ovum matures and travels through the fallopian tube, the endometrium grows and develops in preparation for the embryo. If the ovum is not fertilized in time or if it fails to implant into the endometrium, the arteries of the uterus constrict to cut off blood flow to the endometrium. The lack of blood flow causes cell death in the endometrium and the eventual shedding of tissue in a process known as menstruation. In a normal menstrual cycle, this shedding begins around day 28 and continues into the first few days of the new reproductive cycle.

The menstrual cycle is the monthly cycle of follicle and egg maturation, release of an egg (ovulation), and preparation of the uterine lining for pregnancy. If a woman does not become pregnant, the uterine lining tissue is shed as menstrual bleeding. Most menstrual cycles are 28 days in length. Menarche is the time in during adolescence when menstrual periods begin. Menstrual periods continue to occur until a woman reaches menopause.

* Follicular phase. The follicular phase is the beginning of the menstrual cycle. It starts on the first day of the menstrual cycle and usually lasts about 14 days. The hormones FSH and LH are released from the pituitary gland to stimulate the ovaries. In turn, the ovaries produce estrogen and stimulate the maturation of about 15 to 20 eggs in the ovaries inside small areas known as follicles. Once estrogen levels begin to rise, the secretion of FSH is reduced by a feedback system so that follicle stimulation ceases at the appropriate time. With time, one of the egg follicles (or rarely, two or more) becomes dominant, and maturation of the other follicles is interrupted. The dominant follicle continues to make estrogen.

* Ovulation. Ovulation occurs at the midpoint of the menstrual cycle. Estrogen production from the dominant follicle leads to a sharp rise in LH secretion, causing the dominant follicle to release its egg. The egg is swept into the Fallopian tube by thin structures on the ends of the tubes known as fimbriae. At this time, the cervix produces an increased amount of thick mucus that assists sperm in the passage into the uterus.

* Luteal phase. The luteal phase of the menstrual cycle begins at ovulation (egg release). After the egg is released, the empty follicle turns into a mass of cells called the corpus luteum. The corpus luteum then produces progesterone, a hormone that readies the lining of the uterus for implantation of a fertilized egg. If an egg has been fertilized, the fertilized egg travels down the Fallopian tubes back into the uterus and implants in the uterine lining tissue. If there has not been a fertilization of an egg, the

lining of the uterus eventually breaks down and is shed during menstrual bleeding.

Q. *Is it safe to have sex on my period?*

A. *So you're "calling a code red" and "closing up shop for maintenance" because "mother nature's" calling about her "monthly evacuation" or simply put, you're on your period and you're not feeling so frisky when "Aunt Flo's" in town? Well, you are not alone! Just the mere mention of the words "sex" and "period" in the same sentence, and I don't mean the punctuation mark, can make you feel totally grossed out and leave you cringing in disgust.*

It is common for many women to avoid having sex while on their period. Just the thought of the blood, tampons, maxi pad and fluctuation of hormones can totally ruin the mood. However for some women, having sex while on their period is a natural part of life that comes with many benefits. It is also actually a turn on for many women because estrogen and testosterone start to rise by the third day of the menstrual cycle. Because of this spike in hormones, many women experience a heighten sense of arousal and feel an insatiable desire to be more sexual, and sensual during this time.

Benefits? What benefits?

Having sex during your period can potentially alleviate some of the discomfort of the menstrual cycle. The hormones and endorphins that the body releases during sex, such as oxytocin, helps to relieve mild pain, depression and irritability associated with premenstrual syndrome (PMS). Having sex also increases blood flow which has the potential to minimize headaches and relieve those dreadful cramps. If you're a little on the dry side, menstrual blood actually helps to keep the vagina lubricated which will help to reduce uncomfortable vaginal dryness, ripping and tearing during intercourse. Additionally, with every orgasm, the muscle contractions helps to expel the blood flow and uterine lining much more quickly, thus making your period much shorter. Finally, many women enjoy sex more when they are on their period because of increased feelings of fullness in the pelvic and genitals. This feeling of fullness increase sensitivity and helps with arousal.

With all those benefits to having sex while on your period, why would someone chose not to partake in the pleasures of the period? Hold on—before you decide to get on your "surf board" and take a "ride the crimson wave," there are a few things to take into consideration:

Sexually Transmitted Infection (STI).- *Practicing safer sex is even more essential during your period. Your risks of sexually transmitted diseases and infections are higher than normal during this time because the cervix expands more than usual to allow blood to flow through. This expansion creates a direct pathway for bacteria and viruses to travel deep inside uterus and the pelvic cavity placing a woman at an increased risk for sexually transmitted infections. Also, the vagina has a lower acidity at this time, which puts the female at a greater risk of a yeast or bacterial infection, which also helps to aid in the transmission of STIs, hepatitis and other blood borne diseases. So, on your period or not, safer sex is always the best bet.*

It doesn't feel sexy! *- Due to all the hormonal changes, cramping and bloating, you may not feel sexy or like being intimate during the "time of the month." You may feel unattractive or maybe your partner isn't comfortable with having sex during this time. This is a totally natural feeling. In order to move beyond this feeling, consider taking a hot and steamy shower with your Beloved. Not only will this help to relax you and spice things up but it will also help to reduce any anxieties and concerns about cleanliness. Lots of foreplay will also help to take your mind off of your period and onto your Beloved.*

It can get messy! *- Sex can be messy period, no pun intended. However, if you are concerned, here are a few ways to minimize the mess:*

* *If you're worried about ruining your sheets, having sex on towel will help to take those worries away and keep the sheets clean. You could also turn up your kink meter and consider investing in a pair of rubber sheets.*

* *Having a warm, wet, washcloth or wet wipes nearby to freshen up and quick clean up afterwards can help to reduce the mess.*
* *Your sex positions can also help lessen the mess. Having sex in the missionary position can also limit blood flow. Try to avoid having sex in the female on top because there is the possibility of more leakage due to gravity.*
* *Having sex toward the end of your period, when your flow is lighter, will reduce the likelihood of coming in contact with a lot of blood.*
* *Wearing a digraph, soft menstrual cup or a female condom can help reduce the amount of blood that might come out during intercourse. While these devices may not completely block menstrual flow, they can help absorb some of the blood and/or keep it off of your partner.*
* *If the mess really bothers you, then try having sex in the shower. Since water can dry out the natural lubrication of the vagina, it might be a good idea to also use a silicone-based lubricant.*

It's just nasty! *- Men ejaculate. Women have vaginal fluid and periods. A period is nothing to be afraid of. It is a totally natural, healthy biological process. Menstrual blood, like other bodily fluids, is natural. However, menstrual blood, unlike those other bodily fluids has been stigmatized and considered taboo by society. Historically, female bodies and feminine hygiene have been ostracized and made to feel dirty. Messages received by the media and feminine hygiene companies help to perpetuate this stereotype. In addition, some cultures and religions believe that a woman is unclean during her period. The decision to have sex on while on your period comes down to a personal choice that is based on your comfort level, beliefs and values regarding sexuality and your partner's willingness to indulge.*

I don't have to worry about getting pregnant, right? *- Wrong! There is a chance that you can get pregnant while you're on your period. Although very rare and the likelihood of a woman getting pregnant is very low, it's still not zero. Although every woman's menstrual cycle is different, in general women are usually most fertile about 14 days before the onset of* *their next menstrual period. This is called ovulation. You are likely to get pregnant if you have intercourse a few days before you ovulate, the day you ovulate, and a day or two after you ovulate. Depending on their regularity of their menstrual cycle, some periods last more than a week, some women may ovulate twice a month or even during their period. If you are not on a hormonal birth control method like the pill and are having unprotected sex during this time, there is a possibility of getting pregnant.*

Period sex doesn't only mean intercourse, you've got options! *- So, you and your Beloved have both moved beyond any hesitations about having sex while on your period and you're ready to take things to the next level. Instead of intercourse, allow your partner to earn their "Red Wings" through oral stimulation of the clitoris. To prevent your partner from coming in contact with any fluid that may be coming out of the vagina during this time, be sure to use a dental dam. If you do not have a dental dam, you can use a sheet of plastic wrap or cut a male condom in half and roll it out flat. Remember, oral sex carries the same risk as vaginal and anal sex, so make sure that you always practice safer sex.*

Choosing to have sex during "that time of month" is a personal choice that both you and your Beloved have to be comfortable with. Be informed and understand all the intended and unintended consequences of period sex. Make sure you have the conversation with your partner. Don't surprise your partner in the heat of the moment. Do not be misleading about what's going on with your vagina. Always be upfront and let them in on the decision prior to any sex play. Communication is the key to any sexual experience. As long as your partner is comfortable and you are practicing g safer sex, there's no reason you can't enjoy sexual intimacy at all times, even during your menstrual cycle.

PREGNANCY

If the ovum is fertilized by a sperm cell, the fertilized embryo will implant itself into the endometrium and begin to form an amniotic cavity, umbilical cord, and placenta. For the first 8 weeks, the embryo will develop almost all of the tissues and organs present in the adult before entering the fetal period of development during weeks 9 through 38. During the fetal period, the fetus grows larger and more complex until it is ready to be born. The Pubococcygeus (PC) muscles weaken after childbirth and with age leading to an array of problems such as:

* Accidentally leaking urine when you exercise, laugh, cough or sneeze
* Needing to get to the toilet in a hurry or not making it there in time
* Constantly needing to go to the toilet
* Finding it difficult to empty your bladder or bowel
* Uterus prolapse
* Pain in your pelvic area
* Painful sex

What is the PC muscle?
The PC muscles are attached to the pelvic bone. The function of these muscles is quite similar to that of a hammock—they help to support or hold the pelvic organs together. These muscles are involved with orgasm, sexual pleasure, urine control, fertility, and childbirth. Just as aging, childbearing, gravity, and weight gain result in laxity and sagging of our external muscles, internal muscles are affected as well.

What are the Benefits of Strengthening the PC Muscle?
Kegel exercises are a great way to strengthen the PC muscles. Practicing Kegel exercises help to create direct blood flow to the pelvic floor area, which can have a very positive effect on libido, sexual pleasure, fertility and recovery and tightening post childbearing and into menopause. It is also known to help prevent and treat the incontinence and prolapse health issues. Additionally, strengthened PC muscles lead to orgasming more easily, more frequently and more intensely.

What is the Best Way to Perform Kegel Exercises?

Step 1: Empty your bladder and bowels. Kegel exercises can cause pressure in the pelvic area, which may cause discomfort or an accident if your bladder and bowels are full.

Step 2: Sit or lie in a comfortable position and insert your finger into your vagina. Tighten your vagina around your finger to engage the PC muscle. You should also feel the muscles lift as you squeeze.

Step 3: Relax your muscles and let them drop back into place. Remove your finger.

Step 4: Concentrate on squeezing the muscles without your finger in place. You should feel the same lift and tightening of the walls of the vagina. Breathe normally and avoid tightening your abs or anal muscles.

Step 5: Hold for three seconds and release. Repeat the exercise 10 times.

Step 6: Perform Kegel exercises three times a day. As you become stronger, hold for up to 10 seconds.

Additional Tips for Performing Kegel Exercises:

* If you feel uncomfortable putting your finger in your vagina, you can also locate the PC muscle by stopping the flow of urine. Doing so on a full bladder may weaken the pelvic floor muscles, so only use this method if you are unable to locate the PC muscles another way.

* Kegel exercises may also be performed by using a specially designed tool commonly referred to as "Kegel wand" or "Kegel device."

* Once you become familiar with how the muscles feel when they contract, you can skip steps 2 and 3 and concentrate solely on the Kegel exercises.

A regular use of Kegel exercises works wonders in the sexual life of a woman. It strengthens the vaginal walls to a great extent. This eventually helps a woman to reach more intense and pleasurable orgasms during sexual intercourse. Just as any other muscle, if not exercised, it loses its tone and elasticity and does not perform its function properly.

MENOPAUSE

After child bearing years, a woman begins to enter into menopause. Menopause is a natural part of life. Menopause is defined at the point in time at which a woman has not had a menstrual period for 12 consecutive months. It signals the end of a woman's fertility and occurs, on average, at 51 years of age, but the time of menopause can vary widely. The transition usually has three parts: *perimenopause, menopause,* and *postmenopause.*

Changes usually begin with *perimenopause.* This can begin several years before your last menstrual period. Changing levels of estrogen and progesterone, which are two female hormones made in your ovaries, might lead to symptoms. *Menopause* comes next, the end of your menstrual periods. After a full year without a period, you can say you have been "through menopause," and perimenopause is over. *Postmenopause* follows perimenopause and lasts the rest of your life.

Although menopause signals the end of fertility, you can stay healthy, vital and sexual. Some women feel relieved because they no longer need to worry about pregnancy. Due to the changing levels of estrogen, women may have different signs or symptoms at menopause. As you have less estrogen, some of the most common changes you might notice include hot flashes, low energy, night sweats, sleep problems, mood changes, weight gain, slowed metabolism, thinning hair and dry skin.

If you are having bothersome symptoms, talk to your healthcare provider for help deciding how to best manage menopause. There are many effective treatments are available, from lifestyle adjustments to hormone therapy. Talk with your gynecologist, geriatrician, general practitioner, or internist to help decide what is best for you.

Common Conditions of the Female Reproductive System

"Ouch...that hurts!" is one of the last things you want to say during sex. And pain is definitely not what you want to feel during sex. Not only can it ruin the mood, but it can create significant anxiety around having sex. In addition, it can cause issues within your relationship. Sex is supposed to be pleasurable, not painful. So what happens when it is? If you are experiencing pain during sex, the first step is to try and figure out what's causing the pain. There are a variety of reasons a woman may experience pain during sex. The reasons could be physical and/or psychological. The pain could even be the result of something as simple as the products that you are using irritating the genital area. Knowing what is causing pain is not only crucial to relieving the pain, but also to experiencing pleasure. Here are 10 possible causes:

Dyspareunia

Dyspareunia is recurrent or persistent genital pain before, during, or after sex. It can be acquired, congenital, generalized or situational. Dyspareunia is not a disease, but rather a symptom of an underlying physical, biological or psychological factor. The pain, which is often described as excruciating menstrual cramps, can be mild or severe. It may be superficial, felt in the area around the opening of the vagina and vulva. Or the pain may be deep, felt within the pelvic region or lower back. When the pain occurs, a woman experiencing dyspareunia may be distracted from feeling pleasure and excitement of sex. Due to the persistent experience of pain during sex, a woman still may experience pain during sex even after the original source of pain has disappeared, simply because in her mind, she expects to.

ENDOMETRIOSIS, PELVIC INFLAMMATORY DISEASE (PID), UNDEFINED PELVIC PAIN, FIBROID TUMORS, OVARIAN CYST, CANCER, AND OTHER MEDICAL CONDITIONS

Certain medical conditions may make sex painful because of the scar tissue that forms on internal organs. Not only do these diseases cause pain during sex, but they also adversely affect fertility, diminish quality of life and may cause potentially life-threatening illness. Pelvic pain during intercourse can also result from tears in the ligaments that support the uterus. Regular medical care and treatment of these conditions can help to minimize the effects of these conditions.

LICHEN SCLEROSUS

Lichen sclerosus is an uncommon condition that creates patchy, white skin in the vulva that is thinner than normal. Lichen sclerosus can make sex extremely painful for women due to the itching and scarring. Scarring may narrow the opening of the vagina, which can make penetration painfully difficult. In addition, blistering of the skin may make the vulva unbearable to touch. The exact cause of lichen sclerosus is unknown. However, the condition may be related to a lack of sex hormones. Although lichen sclerosus may involve the skin around the genitals, it is not contagious and cannot be spread through sex.

NEGATIVE BELIEFS, ATTITUDES, BEHAVIORS AND EXPERIENCES WITH SEX

Sex is not only physical—it's emotional, mental and social. The mind and the body works together to optimize the sexual experience. Any negative attitudes, thoughts or beliefs we have been taught regarding sexuality can contribute to uncomfortable sexual experiences. As a result, a woman may experience pain during sex because our bodies are responding to the negative intergenerational patterns, social messages, and misinformation that we have received about sex. In addition, past sexual abuse may subconsciously cause a woman to experience pain during sex. The body's muscle memory may cause the vagina to tense up upon penetration. Even the thought of past sexual trauma can be the source of pain. Psychological factors, emotional stressors, and dissatisfaction in a relationship can decrease sexual responsiveness, and therefore lead to painful intercourse as well.

PRODUCTS THAT YOU ARE USING

Many products contain chemicals that can cause irritation to the vagina and vulva, leading to pain during sex. Some of those products include: contraceptive forms or jellies, latex condoms, vaginal sprays and deodorants, scented tampons, perfumed soaps, laundry detergents and excessive douching. These products can cause the vaginal lining to dry out, making the vagina more prone to rips and tearing during intercourse. In addition, the products can cause inflammation, intense itching and burning to the vulva. Only warm water and a mild soap, if absolutely necessary, should be used to wash the genital area.

> Q. *I heard that douching was not healthy. Can you explain why?*
> A. *The vagina is designed to naturally cleanse itself so there is no need to use a vaginal douche. Additionally, vaginal douching washes away good bacteria that keeps vaginas healthy. Douching also can push bad*

bacteria further up into the reproductive tract, causing infections such as pelvic inflammatory disease, which if left untreated, can cause issues like infertility. Also, steer clear from using perfumed soaps and body washes in the vulva. These products can strip the vulva of its natural oils causing dryness and irritation, creating a portal of entry for STIs and other infections.

VAGINISMUS

Vaginismus is the physical or psychological condition that affects a woman's ability to tolerate vaginal penetration as a result of involuntary vaginal muscle spasms. A woman suffering from vaginismus cannot consciously control the spasm. The vaginismic reflex happens as a result of an object such as a penis, vibrator, tampon, etc. coming towards it. And in some cases, even the thought of the object can cause the vagina to spasm. The involuntary muscle spasm makes penetration painful or impossible. Vaginismus can be either primary or secondary. A woman diagnosed with primary vaginismus has never been able to have penetrative sex or experience vaginal penetration without pain. Secondary vaginismus occurs when a woman who has previously been able to achieve penetration develops vaginismus. The exact cause of vaginismus is unknown; however, it may be due to physical causes, such as an infection or trauma. Some cases of vaginismus may be due to psychological causes, like fear or anxiety. It may also be linked to a combination of causes.

SEXUAL POSITIONS

Certain sexual positions can cause pain during sex. Most positions that allow for deep, thrusting penetration can be painful for a woman, especially if her partner is well endowed or if she has an underlying medical condition. Generally, positions that allow the woman to control the pace and penetration, like woman on top, tend to be more comfortable for a sufferer of painful sex. In order to find out what works, experiment with different positions, techniques and props (i.e. pillows) to find out the one(s) that offer the most stimulation with the least amount of pain.

VULVODYNIA

Vulvodynia is chronic vulvar discomfort or pain, characterized by burning, stinging, irritation or rawness of the female genitalia. In the simplest of terms, vulvodynia means "pain of the vulva." There are two main subtypes of vulvodynia: 1) generalized vulvodynia and 2) vulvar vestibulitis. Generalized vulvodynia is pain that occurs spontaneously and is relatively constant, but there can be some periods of symptom relief. Vulvar vestibulitis syndrome is characterized by pain limited to the vestibule, the area surrounding the opening of the vagina. It occurs during or after pressure is applied to the vestibule. The type of vulvodynia and severity of symptoms experienced are highly individualized. Vulvodynia can have a huge impact on a woman's life. The pain can be so severe that it puts limitations on a woman's ability to function and engage in normal daily activities such as: work, tampon insertion, gynecological exams, sexual relationships and/or physical activities. Most women with vulvodynia feel unable to have sexual intercourse and to fully enjoy life.

YEAST INFECTION

The most common organism that causes yeast infections is known as Candida albicans. This type of yeast can be present in normal, healthy women in the vaginal canal. Most commonly, it is present without causing any symptoms at all. It is only when an overgrowth of this organism is present that symptoms of a yeast infection may manifest. This happens when the balance of protective bacteria in the vagina is disturbed, either due to illness, hormonal changes, or taking certain medications, particularly antibiotics or immune-suppressing drugs. Conditions that affect the function of the immune system, including diabetes, can increase a woman's risk of getting a yeast infection. Sometimes, no cause for the overgrowth of yeast is discovered.

VAGINAL DRYNESS AND LACK OF LUBRICATION

Another frequent explanation for painful sex is thinning and drying of the vaginal tissue. Normally, the lining of the vagina stay lubricated with a thin layer of clear fluid; however, there are many things that can cause the lining to become dry. As the vagina's ability to make its own mucus declines, it becomes irritated, itchy, and painful. Insufficient lubrication or vaginal dryness can cause mild to significant pain and interfere with sexual pleasure. Vaginal dryness is nothing to be embarrassed about. It affects many women, especially as they age. If vaginal dryness begins to affects your lifestyle, sex life and/or relationship with your partner; consider making an appointment with your physician. You do not have to live with uncomfortable vaginal dryness.

> Q. *During intercourse, I get really dry. Half way through the session, it becomes really uncomfortable and sometimes I have to ask my husband to stop. It really frustrates me because I do not understand what's going on. Dr. TaMara, can you please help me with this issue? I mean, I really love my husband and he turns me on, but I do not want him to think he does not because I cannot stay wet.*
>
> A. *Vaginal lubrication is a lubricating fluid that is naturally produced in a woman's vagina. Vaginal lubrication or moistness is always present, but production increases significantly during sexual arousal in anticipation of sexual intercourse.*
>
> *A. thin layer of moisture coats your vaginal walls. When you're sexually aroused, more blood flows to your pelvic organs, creating more lubricating vaginal fluid. Normally, the walls of the vagina stay lubricated with a thin layer of clear fluid, however there are many things that can cause the lining to become dry and irritated. Insufficient lubrication or vaginal*

dryness can cause mild to significant pain (dyspareunia, which is a type of sexual pain disorder) and interfere with sexual pleasure.

WHAT CAUSES DRYNESS?

There are several things that can affect a woman's ability to lubricate, resulting in vaginal dryness. Reduced estrogen levels are the main cause of vaginal dryness. Estrogen helps keep vaginal tissue healthy by maintaining normal vaginal lubrication, tissue elasticity and acidity. These factors create a natural defense against vaginal dryness and infections. But when your estrogen levels decrease, so does this natural defense, leading to a thinner, less elastic and more fragile vaginal lining and an increased risk of infections.

Medical conditions, significant life events, and daily habits such as: pregnancy, lactation, menopause, aging, immune disorders, medical conditions, chemotherapy, sexually transmitted infections, smoking cigarettes, and douching will reduce lubrication and may cause the vagina to feel dry and irritated.

In addition, certain medications will cause dryness, especially those with ingredients that will reduce moisture of the mucosal or "wet" tissues of the vagina. Such medicines include many common drugs for allergies, cardiovascular, psychiatric, and other medical conditions. Oral contraceptives may also decrease vaginal lubrication. Irritation from contraceptive creams and foams can cause dryness, as can fear and anxiety about sexual intimacy.

Vaginal dryness may also result from insufficient foreplay and arousal. In many cases, women need lots of sexual stimulation for arousal. The more aroused she is, the more likely her lubrication will increase; reducing dryness and friction as well as helping to make sexual intercourse more pleasurable.

Vaginal dryness may be accompanied by signs and symptoms such as:

* Itching or stinging around the vaginal opening
* Burning

* Soreness
* Pain with intercourse
* Light bleeding with intercourse
* Urinary frequency or urgency
* Recurrent urinary tract infections
* Involuntary contractions of the pelvic floor muscles

Vaginal dryness is nothing to be embarrassed about. It affects many women, especially as they age. If vaginal dryness begins to affects your lifestyle, sex life and/or relationship with your partner; consider making an appointment with your physician. You don't have to live with uncomfortable vaginal dryness.

WHAT GETS ME WET
Lubricants. Water-based or silicone-based lubricants can help keep your vagina lubricated. Choose products that don't contain glycerin. Glycerin has been linked to yeast infections.

Moisturizers. These products imitate normal vaginal moisture and relieve dryness for up to three days with a single application. Use these as ongoing protection from the irritation of vaginal dryness. Before using complementary or alternative treatments, such as vitamin therapies or products containing estrogen, talk to your physician.

Natural and organic lubricants and cosmetic grade oils such as almond, coconut or olive oils act as lubricants and can be helpful in rejuvenating irritated, dry tissues.

Avoid using these products to treat vaginal dryness because they may dry and irritate your vagina:

* Vinegar, yogurt or other douches
* Hand lotions
* Antibacterial or fragrant soaps
* Bubble baths or bath oils
* Scented or perfumed products

Flavored lubricants are not generally recommended because they can cause a yeast infection. Also, oil-based lubricants are not meant for vaginal use.

Vaginal lubricants can support and/or naturally restore your own vaginal moisture. Whether a woman has an issue or not with lubrication, it is always a good idea to keep lubrication nearby. The more the vagina is lubricated, the less likely the lining of the vaginal will have excessive ripping and tearing from intercourse. Rips and tears in the vaginal help to create a portal of entry for bacteria and other infections. Additionally, please keep in mind that while the use of a lubricant can make sexual intercourse less painful, it does not address the underlying cause of the vaginal dryness itself.

WHAT CAN I DO?

* Pay attention to your sexual needs. Occasional vaginal dryness during intercourse may mean that you aren't sufficiently aroused. Make time for foreplay and allow your body to become adequately aroused and lubricated. Communicate with your Beloved about your sexual needs and what turns you on.
* Having intercourse regularly can also help promote better vaginal lubrication.
* Listen to your body. Vaginal dryness may be an indication that something is going on and you need to go to the physician.
* Boost your water intake. Drinking at least ten 8-oz glasses of water a day may help to relieve vaginal dryness.
* Follow a hormone-balancing diet. Your body needs the right nutritional support to make and balance your hormones.

Finally, just because a woman is wet does not mean that she is ready for sex! It is important to note that there is a difference between arousal and desire. Arousal, which causes lubrication, is physiological and the desire to have sex is psychological. A woman can have the desire to have sex, but not be aroused, which means that there may be some type of is-sue going on that needs to be addressed. In other words, she could want to have sex but her body may not be responding or getting aroused, and vice versa.

A woman's vagina naturally lubricates itself; however, when there is insufficient lubrication, it can cause pain and interfere with sexual pleasure.

When sex hurts, it can definitely dampen the mood, the relation-ship and cause feelings of inadequacy. Please keep in mind that there is a difference between pain and discomfort. Discomfort is a feeling that may not be pleasurable, but it is bearable. Pain is a feeling that is totally unbearable. Pain is an indication that something is wrong with your body and whatever it is that you are doing, you need to stop immediately before you do further damage. If you are experiencing any pain during sex, consider contacting your physician and/or your local sex therapist to get to the root of the problem. Treatment is an option. You do not have to live with unbearable pain forever. Finally, sometimes you might have to get creative and think outside the box when it comes to reducing pain during sex.

Sexually Transmitted Infections

HAVING A SEXUALLY TRANSMITTED INFECTION (STI) can definitely have an impact on sexual pleasure. An STI can cause significant pain to your internal and external sex organs. This pain may intensify during intercourse. STI's can also be pretty tricky. Some STIs, particularly gonorrhea and chlamydia, may not show any symptoms until they cause scarring and major damage to an organ. Additionally, some STIs will cause vaginal itching and dryness which may also make sex pretty painful.

According to the United Sates Department of Health and Human Services, about 19 million new sexually transmitted infections are thought to occur each year. These infections affect women of all backgrounds and economic levels.

There more than 30 different bacteria, viruses, and parasites that can cause an STI. Bacterial STIs include chlamydia, gonorrhea, syphilis, and bacterial vaginosis. Viral STIs include genital herpes, hepatitis B, HPV and HIV. Parasitic STIs include trichomoniasis.

CHLAMYDIA

Chlamydia is one of the most common STIs. It affects approximately 4 million women annually. Because symptoms of chlamydia are not always apparent, it is not easy to tell if a woman is infected with chlamydia.

But when they do occur, they are usually noticeable within one to three weeks of contact and can include the following:

* Vaginal discharge that may have an odor
* Bleeding between periods
* Painful periods
* Abdominal pain with fever pain when having sex
* Itching or burning in or around the vagina
* Pain when urinating

Chlamydia can be detected on material collected by swabbing the cervix during a traditional examination using a speculum. Treatment of chlamydia involves antibiotics. A convenient single-dose therapy for chlamydia is oral azithromycin. However, alternative treatments are often used because of the high cost of this medication. The most common alternative treatment is doxycycline. If left untreated, chlamydia infection can cause pelvic inflammatory disease which can lead to damage of the fallopian tubes (the tubes connecting the ovaries to the uterus) or even cause infertility (the inability to have children). Untreated chlamydia infection could also increase the risk of ectopic pregnancy.

Chlamydia can be cured with the right treatment. It is important that you take all of the medication your doctor prescribes to cure your infection. When taken properly, your medicine will stop the infection and could decrease your chances of having complications later on.

GONORRHEA

Gonorrhea is caused by a bacteria and is one of the oldest known sexually transmitted diseases. It is estimated that over one million women are currently infected with gonorrhea. Among women who are infected, a significant percentage also will be infected with chlamydia. Gonorrhea can only survive on moist surfaces within the body and is found most commonly in the vagina and the cervix. It can also live in the urethra, back of the throat and in the rectum. A majority of infected women have no symptoms, especially in the early stages of the infection. When symptoms do occur, they are usually noticeable within one to three weeks of contact and can include the following:

* Burning or frequent urination
* Yellowish vaginal discharge
* Redness and swelling of the genitals
* Burning or itching of the vaginal area

Like chlamydia, gonorrhea can lead to a severe pelvic infection with inflammation of the fallopian tubes and ovaries, also known as pelvic inflammatory disease (PID).

Testing for gonorrhea is done by swabbing the infected site (rectum, throat, cervix) and identifying the bacteria in the laboratory, either through culturing of the material from the swab (growing the bacteria) or identification of the genetic material from the bacteria. In the past, the treatment of uncomplicated gonorrhea was fairly simple. A single injection of penicillin cured almost every infected person. Unfortunately, there are new strains of gonorrhea that have become resistant to various antibiotics, including penicillin, and are therefore more difficult to treat. Fortunately, gonorrhea can still be treated by other injectable or oral medications. The sexual partners of women who have had either gonorrhea or chlamydia must receive treatment for both infections since their partners may be infected as well. Treating the partners also prevents reinfection of the woman. Women suffering from PID may require more aggressive treatment that is effective against the bacteria that cause gonorrhea as well as against other organisms. These women often require intravenous administration of antibiotics.

Syphilis

Syphilis is an STI that has been around for centuries. It is caused by a bacterial organism called a spirochete. The spirochete is a wormlike, spiral-shaped organism that wiggles vigorously when viewed under a microscope. It infects the person by burrowing into the moist, mucous-covered lining of the mouth or genitals. Symptoms in adults are divided into stages. These stages are primary, secondary, latent, and late syphilis.

Syphilis has been called "the great imitator" because it has so many possible symptoms, many of which look like symptoms from other diseases.

Primary Stage

During the first (primary) stage of syphilis, you may notice only a single sore, but there in fact may be multiple sores. The sore is the location where syphilis entered your body and is usually firm, round, and painless. Because the sore is painless, it can easily go unnoticed. The sore lasts 3 to 6 weeks. In most women, an early infection resolves on its own, even without treatment. Even though the sore goes away, you must still receive treatment so your infection does not move to the secondary stage.

Secondary Stage

During the secondary stage, you may have skin rashes and/or sores in your mouth, vagina, or anus. This stage usually starts with a rash on one or more areas of your body. The rash usually won't itch and it is sometimes so faint that you won't notice it. Other symptoms you may have can include fever, swollen lymph glands, sore throat, patchy hair loss, headaches, weight loss, muscle aches, and fatigue (feeling very tired). The symptoms from this stage will go away whether or not you receive treatment. Without the right treatment, your infection will move to the latent and possibly late stages of syphilis.

The latent stage of syphilis begins when all of the symptoms you had earlier disappear. If you do not receive treatment, you can continue to have syphilis in your body for years without any signs or symptoms. Most people with untreated syphilis do not develop late stage syphilis. However, when it does happen, it is very serious and would occur 10–30 years after your infection began. Symptoms of the late stage of syphilis include difficulty coordinating your muscle movements, paralysis (not able to move certain parts of your body), numbness, blindness, and dementia (mental disorder). In the late stages of syphilis, the disease damages your internal organs and can result in death.

Syphilis can be diagnosed by scraping the base of the ulcer and looking under a special type of microscope (dark field microscope) for the spirochetes. Special blood tests can also be used to diagnose syphilis. The blood tests detect the body's response to the infection, but not to the actual Treponema organism that causes the infection. Syphilis can be cured with the right antibiotics from your health care provider. However, treatment will not undo any damage that the infection has already done.

Depending on the stage of disease, the treatment options for syphilis vary. Penicillin injections have been very effective in treating both early and late stage syphilis. Alternative treatments for syphilis may include oral doxycycline or tetracycline.

BACTERIAL VAGINOSIS

Bacterial vaginosis (BV) is not typically considered to be a sexually-transmitted infection, because some experts feel it can occur in women who are not sexually active. Bacterial vaginosis is the overgrowth or imbalance of certain bacteria within the vagina, leading in some cases to symptoms including a vaginal discharge that may be foul-smelling. Although bacterial vaginosis is found in women of all ages, it is most common vaginal infection in the US in women of childbearing age. Like many other STIs, most women with bacterial vaginosis do not have symptoms from the condition. When symptoms are present, they include abnormal vaginal discharge, fishy odor, vaginal itching and burning, and burning during urination. The best way to diagnose bacterial vaginosis is examination of the vaginal discharge under a microscope by finding a higher than normal vaginal pH and large numbers of bacteria. A pelvic exam, including diagnostic tests for other causes of symptoms, such as gonorrhea and chlamydia, may also be performed at the time of diagnosis. Some of cases of bacterial vaginosis will clear up without any treatment. Nevertheless, treatment with antibiotics is recommended. Metronidazole may be given orally in pill form or applied as a vaginal gel.

Genital Herpes

Genital herpes, also commonly called "herpes," is a viral infection by the herpes simplex virus (HSV) that is transmitted through intimate contact with the mucous-covered linings of the mouth, the vagina or the genital skin. In the United States, about one out of every six people aged 14 to 49 years have genital herpes. The virus enters the linings or skin through microscopic tears. Once inside, the virus travels to the nerve roots near the spinal cord and settles there permanently. When an infected person has a herpes outbreak, the virus travels down the nerve fibers to the site of the original infection. When it reaches the skin, the typical redness and blisters occur. After the initial outbreak, subsequent outbreaks tend to be sporadic. They may occur weekly or even years apart.

Two types of herpes viruses are associated with genital lesions: herpes simplex virus-1 (HSV-1) and herpes simplex virus-2 (HSV-2). HSV-1 more often causes blisters of the mouth area while HSV-2 more often causes genital sores or lesions in the area around the anus. The outbreak of herpes is closely related to the functioning of the immune system. Women who have suppressed immune systems because of stress, infection, or medications, have more frequent and longer-lasting outbreaks.

Genital herpes is spread only by direct person-to-person contact. It is believed that a majority of sexually active adults carry the herpes virus. Part of the reason for the continued high infection rate is that most women infected with the herpes virus do not know that they are infected because they have few or no symptoms.

Once exposed to the virus, there is an incubation period that generally lasts 3 to 7 days before a lesion develops. During this time, there are no symptoms and the virus cannot be transmitted to others. An outbreak usually begins within two weeks of initial infection and manifests as an itching or tingling sensation followed by redness of the skin. Finally, a blister forms. The blisters and subsequent ulcers that form when the blisters break, are usually very painful to touch and may last from 7 days to 2 weeks. The infection is contagious from the time of itching to the time of complete healing of the ulcer, usually within 2 to 4 weeks. However, as noted above, infected individuals can also transmit the virus to their sex partners in the absence of a recognized outbreak.

Only a health care provider can diagnose herpes by performing a physical exam and tests. A blood test can tell if you are infected with oral or genital herpes—even if you don't have symptoms. Genital herpes is suspected when multiple painful blisters occur in a sexually exposed area. During the initial outbreak, fluid from the blisters may be sent to the laboratory to try and culture the virus. There are also blood tests that can detect antibodies to the herpes viruses.

Although there is no known cure for herpes, there are treatments for the outbreaks. Treatments can be are oral medications, such as acyclovir (Zovirax), or topical which are applied directly on the lesions.

Hepatitis B

Hepatitis B virus (HBV) is a virus that causes inflammation of the liver. Most people do not think of hepatitis as a sexually transmitted infection; however, one of the more common modes of the spread of viral hepatitis B is through intimate sexual contact. Hepatitis B is spread through semen, vaginal fluids, blood, and urine. About 46,000 American women, men, and children become infected with HBV each year. Most of these infections occur among people who are age 20 to 49.

Because hepatitis B often has no symptoms, most people are not aware that they have the infection. About 1 out of 2 adults who have it never have hepatitis B symptoms. When hepatitis B symptoms do occur, they usually appear between six weeks and six months after infection. Symptoms most likely to happen first include:

* Extreme tiredness
* Tenderness and pain in the lower abdomen
* Loss of appetite
* Nausea and vomiting
* Pain in the joints
* Headache
* Fever
* Hives
* More severe abdominal pain
* Dark urine
* Pale-colored bowel movements
* Jaundice

Hepatitis B is usually diagnosed by detecting antibodies against the virus and by blood tests that identify the virus in the blood. There is no cure for HBV. HBV usually gets better on its own after a few months. If it does not get better, it is called chronic HBV, which lasts a lifetime. Chronic HBV can lead to scarring of the liver, liver failure, or liver cancer.

Although there is no cure for HBV, it can be treated. Acute hepatitis, unless severe, needs no treatment. Some patients with chronic hepatitis may be treated with antiviral drugs. These medicines can decrease or remove hepatitis B from the blood. They also help to reduce the risk of cirrhosis and liver cancer. If you develop liver failure, a liver transplant is the only cure.

A highly effective vaccine that prevents hepatitis B is currently available. It is recommended that all babies be vaccinated against HBV beginning at birth, and all children under the age of 18 who have not been vaccinated should also receive the vaccination. Among adults, anyone who wishes to do so may receive the vaccine, and it is recommended especially for anyone whose behavior or lifestyle may pose a risk of HBV infection.

HUMAN PAPILLOMAVIRUS (HPV)

HPV infection is now considered to be the most common sexually transmitted infection in the US, and it is believed that at a majority of the reproductive-age population has been infected with sexually transmitted HPV at some point in life. There are more than 40 different types of HPV, types that are transmitted through direct sexual contact, from the skin and mucous membranes of infected people to the skin and mucous membranes of their partners. Some sexually transmitted HPV types may cause genital warts. Persistent infection with "high-risk" HPV types—different from the ones that cause skin warts—may progress to precancerous lesions and invasive cancer. High-risk HPV infection is a cause of nearly all cases of cervical cancer. However, most infections do not cause disease. Most high-risk HPV infections occur without any symptoms, go away within 1 to 2 years, and do not cause cancer. Some HPV infections, however, can persist for many years. Persistent infections with high-risk HPV types can lead to cell changes that if untreated, may progress to cancer.

HPV can sometimes be suspected by changes that appear on a Pap smear, although Pap smears were not really designed to detect HPV. In the case of an abnormal Pap smear, the health care professional will often do advanced testing on the cells to determine if to see if they contain viral DNA or RNA. HPV can also be detected if a biopsy is sent to the laboratory for analysis. An appearance of a genital lesion may prompt the physician to treat without further testing. Genital warts usually appear as small, fleshy, raised bumps, but they can sometimes be extensive and have a cauliflower-like appearance. In many cases genital warts do not cause any symptoms, but they are sometimes associated with itching, burning, or tenderness.

There is currently no medical treatment for persistent HPV infections that are not associated with abnormal cell changes. However, the genital warts, benign respiratory tract tumors, precancerous changes at the cervix, and cancers resulting from HPV infections can be treated.

Currently, there are three vaccines approved to help prevent HPV infection. These vaccines provide strong protection against new HPV infections. HPV vaccination given before sexual activity can reduce the risk of infection by the HPV types targeted by the vaccine. However, they are not effective at treating established HPV infections or disease caused by HPV. In addition, these vaccines are still too new to determine the long-term implications on the body. If you are interested in learning more about the vaccine, talk with your health care professional to determine if the vaccine is right for you.

HUMAN IMMUNODEFICIENCY VIRUS
HIV stands for human immunodeficiency virus.

H: Human—This particular virus can only infect human beings.
I: Immunodeficiency—HIV weakens your immune system by destroying important cells that fight disease and infection. A "deficient" immune system can't protect you.
V: Virus—A virus can only reproduce itself by taking over a cell in the body of its host.

Currently, there is no cure for HIV/AIDS, but there are medications that can dramatically slow disease progression. Once you have HIV, you will have it for life.

What is AIDS?

AIDS stands for Acquired Immune Deficiency Syndrome. To understand what that means, let's break it down:

A: Acquired—AIDS is not something you inherit from your parents. You acquire AIDS after birth.

I: Immune—Your body's immune system includes all the organs and cells that work to fight off infection or disease.

D: Deficiency—You get AIDS when your immune system is "deficient," or isn't working the way it should.

S: Syndrome—A syndrome is a collection of symptoms and signs of disease. AIDS is a syndrome, rather than a single disease, because it is a complex illness with a wide range of complications and symptoms.

Once a person receives a diagnosis of AIDS, it means that he or she has met a predetermined set of criteria as defined by a doctor: if you have one or more specific opportunistic infections or the CD4 cells have fallen below 200. Only a doctor can diagnose someone as having AIDS. CD4 cells are a type of white blood cells that are responsible for protecting the body from infections.

WHAT HAPPENS WHEN HIV ENTERS THE BODY?

When HIV enters the body, it attacks a key part of your immune system—your T-cells, or CD4 cells. HIV invades the cells and uses them to make more copies of itself, and then destroys them. Normally, our body has the ability to fight infections and disease, but a person with a compromised immune system cannot fight off HIV.

During the initial onset or primary/acute infection of HIV, which usually lasts 2-8 weeks, the majority of people develop flu-like symptoms.

Possible signs and symptoms include:

* Fever
* Headache
* Muscle aches
* Rash
* Chills
* Sore throat
* Mouth or genital ulcers
* Swollen lymph glands, mainly on the neck
* Joint pain
* Night sweats
* Diarrhea

Although the symptoms of primary HIV infection may be mild enough to go unnoticed, and undetected on an HIV test, the amount of virus in the bloodstream (viral load) is particularly high at this time and HIV can be spread if an individual is engaging in risky behaviors.

It is important to know that even though the level of the virus may be at a low or undetectable viral load, it does not mean that a person no longer has HIV or that they cannot transmit HIV.

Viral load refers to the amount of HIV in an infected person's blood. An undetectable viral load occurs when the amount of HIV in a person's blood is so low that it can't be measured. However, a person with HIV can still potentially transmit HIV to a partner even if they have an undetectable viral load, because:

* HIV may still be found in a person's genital fluids (e.g., semen, vaginal fluids). The viral load test only measures virus in a person's blood.
* A person's viral load may go up between tests. When this happens, they may be more likely to transmit HIV to partners.

* Sexually transmitted diseases (STDs) increase viral load in a person's genital fluids.

Another particular danger during the initial onset of acute infection period, is that because the signs and symptoms mimic many other conditions, most people either assume they have the flu, treat the signs and symptoms with over-the-counter meds, and/or ignore the symptoms. The danger in this is that they are not tested for HIV unless they know for sure that they have put themselves at risk for HIV.

After the initial onset of acute infection period, the immune system loses the battle with HIV and symptoms go away. HIV infection goes into its second stage, which can be a long period without symptoms, called the asymptomatic, or latent, period. This is when people may not know they are infected and can pass HIV on to others. This period can last 10 or more years. During this period without symptoms, HIV is slowly killing the CD4 T-cells and destroying the immune system.

Over time, HIV destroys so many of the T-cells that the immune system begins to break down. When that happens, HIV infection can lead to the third stage of HIV, an AIDS diagnosis. AIDS is the final stage of HIV infection. However, not everyone who has HIV will progress to AIDS. With proper treatment and maintaining medical adherence, an individual infected with HIV can keep the level of HIV in their body low.

WHAT ARE THE FLUIDS THAT TRANSMIT HIV?

HIV is transmitted by coming in contact with certain body fluids of a person that is infected with HIV. These body fluids are:

* Blood
* Semen (cum)
* Pre-seminal fluid (pre-cum)
* Vaginal fluids
* Breast milk

These body fluids must come into contact with a mucous membrane or damaged tissue or be directly injected into your bloodstream (by a needle or syringe) for transmission to possibly occur. Mucous membranes are the soft, moist areas just inside the openings to your body such as inside the rectum, the vagina, the opening of the penis, and the mouth.

HIV is most commonly diagnosed by testing your blood or saliva for antibodies and/or the virus. Most people who get tested for HIV will show an accurate result after about two to eight weeks from infection. In rare cases, it may take up to six months for enough HIV antibodies to build up in the blood to be detected on an HIV antibody test. Currently, there is no cure for HIV—only treatment. Early HIV antiretroviral treatment is crucial—it improves quality of life, extends life expectancy and reduces the risk of transmission.

TRICHOMONIASIS
Trichomoniasis, sometimes referred to as "trich," is a common STD that affects 2 to 3 million Americans yearly. It is caused by a single-celled protozoan parasite called trichomonas vaginalis. Trichomoniasis is primarily an infection of the urogenital tract; the urethra is the most common site of infection in man, and the vagina is the most common site of infection in women. Trichomoniasis, like many other STIs, often occurs without any symptoms. When and if symptoms appear, usually within four to 20 days of exposure, they include:

* Heavy, yellow-green or gray vaginal discharge
* Discomfort during intercourse
* Vaginal odor
* Painful urination
* Abdominal pain
* Vaginal itching and irritation
* Painful sex

Trichomoniasis is usually diagnosed by a physical examination and lab test. Lab tests are performed on a sample of vaginal fluid or urethral fluid to look for the disease-causing parasite.

The oral antibiotic metronidazole is used to treat women with trichomoniasis. It usually is administered orally in a single dose. Your partner should also be treated at the same time to prevent reinfection and further spread of the disease. In addition, persons being treated for trichomoniasis should avoid sex until they and their sex partners complete treatment and have no symptoms. It is important to take all of your antibiotics, even if you feel better.

If you suspect that you have an STI, it is important to be evaluated as soon as possible to relieve the pain and/or reduce the chances of infertility.

How Can I Protect Myself From STIs?

WHEN YOU ENTER INTO A sexual relationship, it is extremely important that you take the time to get to know your sexual partner. Failure to do so may result in dire consequences, like becoming infected with HIV and other sexually transmitted infections. Taking the following precautions when beginning a sexual relationship can help reduce your likelihood of becoming infected.

LET'S TALK CONDOMS AND DENTAL DAMS

How many times have you heard, "it doesn't feel good with a condom", "just let me put the tip in", or "I promise I'll pull out?" Have you ever thought that each and every time you have sex without a condom, it is like playing Russian roulette? You may dodge the HIV bullet, or you may not. Just like bullets, HIV does not discriminate. You also have to consider that if your partner will have unprotected sex with you, then he or she is also likely to have unprotected sex with others. Keep in mind that every time you have sex, unprotected or not, you're having sex with everyone that they have had sex with. Now just imagine how many people you have theoretically shared body fluids with. When used correctly and consistently, condoms offer the best protection against HIV and STIs.

FEMALE CONDOM

Women are becoming more empowered and proactive in taking control of their sexual health. It is no longer considered the man's responsibility to pull out a condom, or even put it on, during sex play. In the past, sexual norms, negative intergenerational patterns, gender roles and inequalities, lack of access to resources, lack of communication skills and low self-esteem have all put women at a greater risk of contracting HIV and other sexually transmitted infections. In addition, because messages about female sexuality in our society have been so over-sexualized yet taboo and stigmatized, many women have not received comprehensive sex education or sex positive messages regarding their sexuality. Furthermore, the idea of purchasing and/or carrying condoms have been judged and condemned with messages that "good girls don't, only fast girls do," "sex before marriage is immoral" and/or "if you have sex, you're loose, a whore or a slut." All of these factors contribute to increasing vulnerability, which unfortunately makes women more powerless to protecting themselves in sexual situations.

Well, now it's time to transform judgment into love, do away with labels, dispel myths and start replacing them with messages of empowerment so that women can begin to be more responsible in protecting themselves. The female condom is a great way for women to take the sexual responsibility into their own hands.

The female condom is a pouch with flexible rings at each end. Before vaginal intercourse, the ring inside the pouch is inserted deep into the vagina, holding the condom in the vagina. The penis is directed into the pouch through the ring at the open end, which stays outside the vaginal opening during intercourse. *Warning: Female condoms and male condoms cannot be worn at the same time. The friction of intercourse will cause both condoms to break...which defeats the purpose.*

Additional benefits of the female condom include:

* Women can still protect themselves even if their partner refuses to wear a condom

- Women can insert a female condom for up to 6 hours before intercourse, so it doesn't interfere with the "heat of the moment"
- The female condom can be used if one or both parties have an allergy to latex
- The female condom is available over the counter without a prescription
- The female condom offers additional protection as compared to the male condom because it covers the labia or the "lips" of the vagina
- Because the female condom is made of polyurethane, which is a slightly thicker rubber than latex, it creates a warming sensation during sex

A little to trick to enhance sensation for the male partner is to place a little water-based or silicone-based lubricant inside of the female condom. This will provide more sensation for him.

Carrying condoms—male or female—does not make a woman promiscuous, no more so than does purchasing automobile insurance means that you are going to get into an accident! A woman who carries condoms is a woman who is smart enough to have the necessary "insurance" in place to protect herself just in case she finds herself in a sexual situation. The female condom definitely gives women the means and the power to protect themselves without having to rely on their partner. In this day and age, it is extremely important for women to have the knowledge, skills and tools necessary to facilitate safer and more pleasurable sexual experiences! At the end of the day, we are responsible for our own sexual health, so YES… women should carry condoms too.

MALE CONDOM

"Oh #@%! The condom broke!"—a phrase you never want to hear during the midst of sex play! Talking about a mood killer! What?! The penis immediately goes south, the once plentiful flowing waters of the vagina instantly dry up like a barren desert and the look of anxiety replaces the sex face of passion because now you're effectively terrified of the unintended consequences of unprotected sex.

Before we go further, here are a few facts. If used correctly and consistently each time, condoms are 98-100% effective and offer the best protection against most sexually transmitted infections (STI) and unintended pregnancies. But even at 98-100% rate of effectiveness, studies show that condoms have a 2% rate of failure with the most common cause due to inconsistent usage, breakage and/or misuse. Most commonly, condom mishaps or breakage occurs when the user fails to follow the steps for using and putting on a condom properly. Right now, you're probably saying to yourself, "There are steps for using a condom?" YES, there are steps and most manufacturers have written instructions! And, knowing the proper steps for putting on a condom can significantly reduce the chances of breakage, slippage, unintended pregnancies and transmission of most STIs; however, many people are unaware or have been misinformed.

STEPS FOR PUTTING ON A CONDOM:
Here are the recommended steps for using condoms before and during sex play, each and every time.

1. Check the expiration date printed on the individual package. If expired, do not use. Only use unexpired condoms!
2. Squeeze the condom package to ensure that the package is properly sealed. All of sides and edges should be sealed tight, the package should have no punctures or holes and a bubble of air is usually trapped in the center of the package.
3. When opening the package, push condom to the side and open the package using your index finger tips and thumbs. Do not use your teeth, fingernails or sharp tools to open package as this may puncture the condom.
4. Pull condom out of the package with your index finger and thumb.

5. Before applying to the penis, make sure the tip of the condom is facing upward. Pinch the tip with the fingertips of one hand while unrolling the condom all the way down from the top to the base of the penis with the fingertips of the other hand.
6. Once the sperm has been released, immediately pull the penis and condom out of your partner.
7. To remove the condom, pull from the tip and pushing from the base (may require both hands)
8. Wrap the used condom into a disposal tissue and properly discard.

Q. *I just noticed that every time I have sex with a condom, my vagina is itchy and irritated? Could there be something wrong with the condoms I am using?*

A. *There is a possibility that you may have a latex allergy. If that is the case, stay away from the latex! The irritation that you experience can make you more susceptible to infections. You may consider trying to use a polyurethane and polyisoprene condom. They provide a fantastic alternative to latex. An added advantage to polyisoprene condoms is that they're ultra-thin, which offers a more natural feel!*

FACTS ABOUT CONDOMS

Making the decision not to wear a condom is like playing a game of Russian roulette —you never know when the bullet will hit you. Avoid the condom "cock blocking" at all cost!

"But I don't like using a condom!"
"I can't feel it!"
"I want to feel the REAL you!"
"My dick gets soft when I put on a condom!"
"What...you don't trust me? I'm clean!"

Just a few of the not-so-clever excuses one uses when it comes to condom aversion. Stop with the excuses and wrap it up! Would you rather find yourself explaining to a doctor why you have an itching a burning sensation with an icky drip coming from your penis, or perhaps why you have a foul smelling discharge coming from your vagina? I think not! In lieu of abstinence, condoms are the best protection we have against STIs! In order to be effective, condoms should be used consistently and correctly for anal, oral or vaginal sex. Condoms should only be used with a water-based or silicone-based lubricant, as this helps to reduce friction and chances of the condom breaking. DO NOT use any oil based lubricants such as: massage oils, vegetable oil, Vaseline or motor oil. The oil will break down a condom in less than 60 seconds and put you at risk.

<u>Here are some important things to know:</u>

1. All men don't wear Magnums! Condoms come in sizes ranging from snuggies to extra-large! There is no one size fits all, although one size fits most! Nevertheless, it's still important to get the proper size for your manhood. The importance of wearing the proper size condom is essential to the level of protection. Wearing the wrong size condom can also increase the chance of breaking and slippage. If for example the condom is too large, it is more likely to slip off during intercourse. If the condom is too small, it can actually burst during intercourse. In either case, you've defeated your purpose for putting the condom on.

2. Variety is the spice of Life! BCondoms, Trojan, LifeStyles, Durex, Trustex, Beyond Seven, Kimoto...with so many condom brands on the market, how does one choose? What's the best condom to use? The best condom to use is the one that works the best for you and your partner(s). Condoms come in all different brands, textures, flavors and styles. Ribbed, studded, contoured, French Tickler,

extra pouch, all of which are designed to enhance pleasure. You and your partner should take advantage of this and explore until you find the condom brand, texture and style that fits your needs! Condoms also come in a variety of flavors to suit your taste buds. Flavored condoms should only be used for oral sex and not vaginal sex because flavored condoms have glycerin, a sugar in the flavoring, the potential for yeast infections increases if used vaginally. Turn your search for the "perfect" condom into a game that you and your Beloved can play together as you explore and try out different brands until you find the one that you like best!

3. My partner is allergic to latex, so I can't use a condom. Ah! But you can! Polyisoprene and polyurethane condoms are specially made for those who have a latex allergy. Both condoms are made of a different type of rubber that reduces the chances of irritation and allergic reaction that some women and men will experience from latex. Also, both the polyisoprene and polyurethane condoms are just as effective as the latex condom and provide the same level of protection.

4. I heard that lambskin condoms have a more natural feel. Stay away from the lambskin condoms! Lambskin condoms are only good for prevention of pregnancy—they are ineffective for protection against HIV and other STIs. This is because lambskin condoms are made of sheep/lamb intestines which, much like our intestines, have pores. The molecular structures of STIs are so small that it can seep through the pores of the lambskin condom, consequently putting you at risk for sexually transmitted infections.

5. Store condoms in a cool, dry place (below 100° F), not in the glove box or in your pocket and avoid exposure to direct sunlight. If latex is sticky or brittle when removed from package, do not use the condom. Condoms should be stored in a location i.e. dresser drawer, nightstand, "toy box," etc. that makes them easily accessible.

Additional Tips:

- Never go from anal sex to vaginal sex using the same condom. If you do, you are increasing your possibility of getting an infection.
- Avoid using novelty condoms, such as glow in the dark condoms. Novelty condoms are just that, novelties. They are not intended for use in sexual activity.
- Condoms clog toilets! Don't flush any condom down the toilet. Throw away it in trashcan.
- Never use a condom more than once.
- If the color of the condom is changed or uneven, do not use. If you have multiple partners, use a new condom with each one.
- Condoms can also be used with sex toys, such as vibrators and dildos, to reduce risk of infection.

NOW LET'S TALK ABOUT DENTAL DAMS...

What on earth is a dental dam, Dr. TaMara? A dental damn is a thin, square sheet of latex or polyurethane used for oral-vaginal sex and oral-anal sex to help prevent the person's mouth from coming in contact with any bodily fluids.

During oral sex, dental dams should be placed between your mouth and the vagina. During anal sex, dental dams are placed between your mouth and the anus.

Dental dams should only be used one time and on one area of the body before being thrown away. You should never flip (or turn over) already used dental dams because that could result in the exchange of body fluids. Dental dams can also be used with lubricants for increased sensation. You can also put a bit of lubricant (that isn't oil based) on the side of the dental dam that touches the skin to keep the latex from sticking. Dental dams also come in a variety of glycerin free flavors to help with the taste.

Dental dams can be purchased from drugstores, online, community based organizations or AIDS service organization and from various public health departments. Unfortunately though, many people report that dental dams may be hard to find, and they can also be somewhat expensive. The good news is that dental dams are easy to make at home—all you need is a condom and scissors. So how do you make a dental dam?

To Make Dental Dams:

1. Unroll a condom
2. Cut off the tip very carefully
3. Cut down one side of the condom
4. Roll it out flat

When making your own dental dams, it may be better to use a non-lubricated latex condom (as condoms lubricated with spermicide may taste bad or make your tongue numb). You can also choose to make dental dams from flavored condoms or from condoms and lubricants designed specifically for use during oral sex.

BEYOND CONDOMS AND DENTAL DAMS, HERE ARE SOME ADDITIONAL WAYS TO PROTECT YOURSELF!

In lieu of abstinence, condoms and dental dams are the best protection we have against STIs! In order to be effective, condoms should be used consistently and correctly for anal, oral or vaginal sex. When used consistently and correctly, barrier methods are very effective in STI and HIV prevention; however, here are some alternative ways to protect yourself:

Get tested for HIV together. If you and your Beloved are serious about taking your relationship to a sexual level, then consider going to get tested for HIV together. More importantly, go back to get your results together. When getting tested for HIV, you may also want to consider getting tested for other STIs. Some STIs, such as chlamydia and gonorrhea are asymptomatic and may go undetected. Additionally, if a person has an STI, he or she is five times more likely to get HIV. While getting tested is great, it should not be your method of prevention. Changing behaviors that put you at risk for HIV, open and honest communication, and mutual monogamy should be your goal.

Identify triggers. It is very important to learn what triggers your sexual responsiveness. For example, if you know that when you go out to the club, you're likely to have a few drinks and end up leaving with someone to have sex, then the club is a trigger that you need to avoid and replace with a more healthy activity. Learning to identify what gets your hormones raging is essential to learning how to avoid those triggers and reduce your risk for HIV and other STIs.

Change the type of sex you are having. Variety is the spice of life and we all like to break the monotony in the bedroom, or where you're having sex. However, the types of sex we're having may be contributing to one's risk for HIV. Changing the type of sex you're having will also help to reduce your risk. Anal sex carries the most risk because the lining of the anus is thin and does not lubricate naturally, causing it to rip and tear much easier. Vaginal sex is the second most risky type of sex, followed by oral sex. Keep in mind that the receptive partner is the partner that is most at risk because she or he is receiving the penis inside their anus or vagina. This increases their risk given the exposure to the fluid. Here's an FYI about oral sex—do not brush or floss or participate in any activity that can cause a tear or break in the lining of the jaw an hour or less before oral sex, because it will actually increase the risk for HIV transmission. If any semen or vaginal fluid gets inside of your mouth, swallow, spit but don't let it sit!

Reduce the number of sexual partners. If you are a person that likes to engage in sex with multiple partners, keep in mind that also puts you at higher risks, especially if the encounters are unprotected. Think of it this way, every time you have sex with someone, you're having sex with everyone that they have had sex with. Not only does reducing the number of sexual partners lower your risk for HIV, but it also lowers your risk for drama and other indirect activities that put you at risk for HIV and other STIs.

Hold up on the substances. We all have brought into the belief that alcohol makes the sex better—heck, Jamie Foxx even sung a song about it blaming it on the alcohol. However, substances, no matter what the type, actually put you at an increased risk for HIV and other sexually transmitted infections. Anytime we over-indulge in substances, our mental state becomes altered. Impaired judgement causes you to make decisions that you would not normally make, such as having casual sexual encounters because your hormones are turned up. Substances can also impair motor skills that inhibit your ability to put on a condom and/or dental; that is, if you can even think through the haze of your buzz to use one. In addition, substances can contribute to erectile issues in men and vaginal dryness in women, which can contribute to more ripping and tearing during intercourse, creating a portal of entry for infections to inter the bloodstream.

Take time to get to know your partner. What's the rush? Casual sex does not come without a cost and the cost could just be your life. Be sure to ask questions. With every sexual encounter, you must ask yourself if this orgasm is worth my life and am I willing to die for sex? Because that's what you are essentially saying when you fail to ask your sexual partners questions about their sexual past. Everyone has a sexual history. While the *number* of partners isn't that important (because most people won't be honest anyway), you should be more concerned with if he or she has had safer sex during **every single** sexual encounter. Additionally, questions to ask include: Have you been tested for HIV? Did you get your results? What were your results? Have you ever had a STI? If so, did you get it treated? For heterosexual-identified individuals, you may also consider asking if your partner has ever engaged in any same-sex sexual tryst? For lesbian or gay identified individuals, you may want to ask if they have ever had sex with someone of the opposite sex. As difficult as it may be to ask these questions, it is very important to ask your sex partners about their sexual past. At the end of the day, if you cannot ask your partner these questions, then maybe you should not be having sex with them.

Turn the lights on and open your eyes! Let's say that you do not want to turn the lights on because you're concerned how your body looks or you want to be romantic. While having sex with the lights off can be less intimidating or be romantic, it can also be very dangerous. It is time to stop flipping the switch and turn the light on and look at what you are getting yourself into. FYI, male condoms do not cover the testicles, vulva, or the perineum, so if there are any genital warts or herpes lesions on any of those areas, you may be putting yourself at risk for transmission. In addition, you need to look at your sex partner's genitals to notice if there is any abnormal discharge coming out of the vagina or penis. If the lights are off and/or if you are not looking at your sex partner, then how can you keep yourself safer? Finally, when a person has one STI, it makes it much easier for them to get another—like five times easier! Do not become a statistic because you are in the dark with your eyes closed.

Learn to abstain. Your body is a temple! Everyone does not deserve to receive your most precious gift. When you know your value and worth, you're less likely to do things to put yourself in danger. You respect yourself and your body, and you are very cautious about whom you share yourself with. Every time you have sex with someone, you give a piece of yourself away that you cannot get back. There is an exchange of energy that remains with you; therefore, it is extremely critical that you are protective of the energy that you allow inside of your being. Finally, abstaining means also avoiding those "triggers" and substances that help to put an individual at risk for transmission of HIV/STIs.

Take control of your sexuality. Don't allow love or your hormones to get the best of you. Make wise decisions regarding your sexual health. Remember, you are responsible for your sexual health. Women are sexually empowered and liberated, but being sexually empowerment and liberated does not mean loose—it means being in control of your sexuality, which includes your sexual desires and sexual expressions.

Practice sexual exclusivity. Sexual exclusivity is similar to monogamy, in that it involves making the conscious decision to engage in sexual activities with only one person, regardless of whether or not you are in a coupled relationship. By practicing sexual exclusivity, you are reducing the number of sexual partners, which helps to lower risk for STIs and HIV.

Don't forget about the lube. Wetter is better, especially when it comes to sex. Vaginal lubrication is key to sexual pleasure for both men and women. Lubricant comes in a few forms: water-based, silicone-based and oil-based. Water- and silicone-based lubes are the best with condoms. Never use an oil-based lubricant with a condom—the oil will interact with the latex and cause it to break down. A good lubricant can go a long way in making sure that safer sex is pleasurable and fun. Lubricant is important in safer sex because it also makes condoms and dams slippery and less likely to break. Lubricants make safer sex feel better by cutting down on the dry kind of friction that a lot of people find irritating.

At the end of the day, you have to ask yourself if that 5 or 10 minutes of pleasure is worth your life? HIV is real! Although a person can live with HIV for several years, the quality of life can be greatly reduced. And while the individual is infected, the family, and community is affected. Don't allow love or your hormones to get the best of you. Take time to protect yourself. You are responsible for your sexual health. It's important to get tested, know your status, change behaviors, and build skills. This will help to reduce your risk for becoming infected with HIV. Finally, I leave you with this—every time you have unprotected sex with someone whose HIV or STI status you do not know, you are saying to them, "I love you enough to let you kill me!" Ask yourself one simple question: is this ten, fifteen maybe twenty minutes of pleasure worth dying for? I think NOT! Respect yourself enough to protect yourself! Wrap it up! Safer sex is the new sexy!

<u>*Pearls of Wisdom*</u>: *Making Safer Sex Sexy*

* *Safer sex begins with you! Be comfortable with who you are as a sexual being and your sexuality! You cannot truly share your sexuality if you are not comfortable with who you are. Certainly, if you're not comfortable with who you are, you cannot talk to or teach anyone to be comfortable with their sexuality. In addition, you cannot negotiate safer sex if you are not comfortable with your sexual self, nor can you talk to your physician about your sexual health.*

* *Add toys to the mix. Anything by "Bedroom Kandi" will definitely enhance the experience! (Bedroom Kandi is an intimate luxury adult product line of Grammy Award Winning Songwriter/Producer & TV star Kandi Burruss.)*

* *Eroticize the condom by putting it on with your mouth. He'll more than likely be so amazed that you can actually do it that he would be more than willing to let you try!*

* *Build anticipation and intensify the experience by playing lover's games.*

* *Mutual masturbation is a great way to share the sexual experience while lowering your risk for HIV and other STIs. The visual of your partner masturbating can be very erotic and arousing for some.*

* *Use flavored lubricants. You can purchase lubricants in a variety of flavors, from spicy to sweet; there are options for the chocoholics out there, too. Some cause warming sensations, some make you tingle, and if you're looking for an icy blast, pick up a cooling lube. However, I caution you to make sure to use glycerin-free flavored lubes.*

* *Get out of the bedroom. The bedroom is for sleeping. Add a little bit of naughtiness to your sex life by trying out new locations for your sexual trysts.*

- *Share fantasies and role play. Doing so helps to increase communication and intimacy when you share your sexual fantasies with your Beloved. Besides, you're unlikely to be distracted about whether or not a condom feels good when your partner is dressed up in something sexy.*
- *Focus on pleasure and intimacy. Sex isn't always about penetration. Don't be in such a rush to have intercourse. Take time to explore each other bodies.*
- *Try a variety of condoms. With all the different types and brands of condoms on the market, this could literally go on forever!*
- *Create a safer sex kit. Go shopping together. Talk about what you each want and need to feel safe. Make a sex kit that is just for the two of you, creating a cool case or container that's personalized. If you don't like the brand of condom or lube you're using, explore together to find what does work best for the both of you. You can make a date out of STI testing instead of going it alone. When you and your partners share responsibilities with sex, caring well for one another mutually, it can not only keep you both healthy so you can enjoy that relationship best, it can deepen your bond and your partnership.*
- *Change your perspective. One of the most important aspects of introducing a new routine into your sex life is looking at it in a positive context. Think about safer sex products as a kind of permission slip; once you put it on, you can now relax and enjoy your sexual escapades knowing that you have taken the best possible precautions against unwanted incidents. Peace of mind can be a great turn-on!*

Routine Testing and Screenings Every Woman Should Have

PELVIC EXAM

The word "pelvic" refers to the pelvis. A pelvic exam helps a health care professional evaluate the size and position of the vulva, uterus, cervix, fallopian tubes, ovaries, bladder and rectum.

A pelvic exam may be done to also help detect certain cancers in their early stages, infections, including sexually transmitted infections (STIs), or other reproductive system problems.

Pelvic exams are usually performed during a routine yearly physical exam, when a woman is pregnant, when a doctor is checking for an infection, and/or when a woman is having pain in her pelvic area or low back. Pelvic exams may also be used to determine the cause of abnormal uterine bleeding, evaluate pelvic organ abnormalities, such as uterine fibroids, ovarian cysts, or uterine prolapse and to collect evidence in cases of suspected sexual assault. Finally, a health care professional may conduct a pelvic exam before prescribing a method of birth control (contraception). Some methods of birth control, such as a diaphragm or intrauterine device, require a pelvic exam to make sure the device fits properly.

During a pelvic exam, you can expect to feel a little discomfort, but you should not feel pain during a pelvic exam. The exam itself takes about 10 minutes. If you have any questions during the exam, be sure to ask your doctor. A Pap test may also be done during the pelvic exam.

During a typical pelvic exam, your doctor or nurse will:

* Talk to you about any health concerns.
* Ask you to take off your clothes in private (You will be given a gown or other covering.)
* Ask you to lie on your back and relax.
* Press down on areas of the lower stomach to feel the organs from the outside
* Help you get in position for the speculum exam (You may be asked to slide down to the end of the table.)
* Ask you to bend your knees and to place your feet in holders called stirrups.
* Perform the speculum exam. During the exam, a device called a speculum will be inserted into the vagina. The speculum is opened to widen the vagina so that the vagina and cervix can be seen.
* Perform a Pap smear. Your doctor will use a plastic spatula and small brush to take a sample of cells from the cervix (A sample of fluid also may be taken from the vagina to test for infection.)
* Remove the speculum.
* Perform a bimanual exam. Your doctor will place two fingers inside the vagina and uses the other hand to gently press down on the area he or she is feeling. Your doctor will note if the organs have changed in size or shape.
* Sometimes a rectal exam is performed. Your doctor inserts a gloved finger into the rectum to detect any tumors or other abnormalities.
* Talk to you about the exam (You may be asked to return to get test results.)

When scheduling a pelvic exam, try to schedule the exam when you are not on your menstrual cycle, since blood can interfere with the results of a Pap test. However, if you have a new vaginal discharge or new or increasing pelvic pain, a pelvic exam may be done while you are having your period. Do not use douches, tampons, vaginal medicines, or vaginal sprays or powders for at least 24 hours. Do not have sex for 24 hours prior to the exam if you have abnormal vaginal discharge. No other special preparations are needed before having a pelvic exam. For your own comfort, you may want to empty your bladder before the exam.

If you have had problems with pelvic exams in the past or have experienced rape or sexual abuse, be sure to talk with your health care professional about your concerns or fears before the exam.

PAP TEST

A Pap test, sometimes referred to as a Pap smear, is a method of cervical screening used to detect abnormalities in the cervical cells that may be potentially pre-cancerous and/or cancerous. Currently, a pap test is the best tool to detect precancerous conditions and hidden, small tumors that may lead to cervical cancer. If detected early, cervical cancer can be cured. Women should begin routine pap testing at the age of 18 or at the onset of sexual activity, if earlier, and continue screenings annually. After three or more consecutive satisfactory normal annual exams, the Pap test may be performed less frequently at the discretion of your health care professional. Screenings may be stopped for women over the age of 65 who have been adequately screened with normal results in the last 10 years and are not at high risk for cervical cancer. Most women ages 21 to 65 should get Pap tests as part of routine health care. Even if you are not currently sexually active, you should still have a Pap test. Women who do not have a cervix (usually because of a hysterectomy), and who also do not have a history of cervical cancer or abnormal Pap results do not need Pap tests.

The Pap test is normally done during a pelvic exam. A doctor uses a device called a speculum to widen the opening of the vagina so that the cervix and vagina can be examined. A plastic spatula and small brush are used to collect cells from the cervix. After the cells are taken, they are placed into a solution. The solution is sent to a lab for testing.

A normal Pap test means the cells from the cervix look normal. An abnormal Pap test means the cells do not look normal. In that case, further testing may need to be done to determine the cause for the abnormality, i.e. cervical dysplasia. Pap tests can occasionally show signs of infection but cannot be relied on to screen for sexually transmitted infections (STIs). Other tests are necessary to determine the presence of an STI.

There are several things you can do to help make the Pap test as accurate as possible. These include avoidance of sex, douching, and vaginal creams for 48 hours before the test. In addition, do not schedule a Pap test during your menstrual cycle. The best time to be tested is 10 to 20 days after the first day of your period.

Regular Pap test screening, early detection and treatment of abnormal cervical cells is critical tool in finding and treating cervical cell changes before they progress to cervical cancer. If cervical cancer is suspected, your health care professional will proceed with additional testing.

BREAST EXAM

Women should begin examining their breasts once a month at or around the age of 20. Examining the breasts regularly allows a woman to be aware of what feels natural and what does not. Any unusual breast symptoms or changes in the breast tissue such as: swelling, dimpling, nipple discharge, persistent pain, redness, unusual masses or any other variation in how the breast looks and feels should be reported immediately to your health care professional. It is important to following current guidelines and recommendations for screenings.

Breast exam can be performed by your physician as a part of your routine annual exam, which also includes your pelvic exam and PAP Test. Between annual exams, you should also be performing your own breast self-exam (BSE). If it is your first time performing s BSE, your physician can show you the most effective way to perform your exam.

The most effective way to detect breast cancer is by mammography, and a clinical breast exam can complement mammography screening.

* Mammogram: Beginning at age 40, every woman should have a mammogram once every one to two years, or more frequently if breast cancer runs in her family. A mammogram produces images of the inner breast tissue using a very low dose of radiation produced by a machine specifically designed for mammograms. Mammograms can help identify cysts, calcifications and tumors within the breast. It is currently the most effective way to detect early breast cancer.
* Clinical breast exam by a trained health care professional: Clinical breast exams should begin at age 20 and be repeated every three years until age 40. For women over 40, exams should continue annually. During a clinical breast exam, a health care professional will visually and manually examine the breasts for anything abnormal, such as: swelling, dimpling, nipple discharge, persistent pain, redness, unusual masses and any other variation in how the breasts look and feel. If she or he detects any abnormality during the exam, then they may refer the patient for a more in-depth screening such as a mammogram.

Pearls of Wisdom: If you have breast implants, it may be useful to have your surgeon or doctor assist you in identifying the edges of the implants so you can identify any changes you may feel in your breasts.

SEXUALLY TRANSMITTED INFECTION (STI) SCREENING

Most people think they would know if they had a sexually transmitted infection (STI)...wrong! The truth is that many STIs have no signs or symptoms in the majority of people infected, or they have mild signs that can be easily overlooked. This is why the term "disease" (as in STD) is starting to be replaced by "infection" (or STI). Because some STIs are asymptomatic, it is important for an individual to be tested for STIs if there has been a risk of exposure, even if they do not have symptoms. The only way to know if you have an STI is to get tested.

Although STI tests can be performed during an annual gynecological exam, this is not always done. Some providers might test for some infections when you come in for a regular check-up, while others do not test for any STI unless you ask them to.

The most common STIs are chlamydia, gonorrhea, HIV, herpes, HPV, syphilis and trichomoniasis. Getting tested for an STI can be quick and easy. Depending on what you are being tested for, your health care professional may take a physical exam, blood sample, a swab, or urine sample. If you believe that you have been exposed to an STI, talk to your healthcare professional about getting tested. Getting tested can put your mind at ease and get you (and your partner) treatment. It is also important to learn about ways you and your partner can protect yourselves in the future through safer sex.

HIV Test

Current CDC guidelines recommend that that individuals aged 13-64 get tested at least once in their lifetimes and those with risk factors, direct and indirect, get tested more frequently. HIV is most commonly diagnosed by testing your blood or saliva for antibodies and/or the virus.

Most people who get tested for HIV will show an accurate result after about two to eight weeks from infection. In rare cases, it may take up to six months for enough HIV antibodies to build up in the blood and be detected on an HIV antibody test.

While it is important to get tested for HIV, it is more important go back and get your results together. When getting tested for HIV, you may also want to consider getting tested for other STIs. Some STIs, such as chlamydia and gonorrhea are asymptomatic and may go undetected. Additionally, if a person has an STI, he or she is five times more likely to get HIV.

HIV testing is the only way to determine if you are infected with HIV. Most individuals who are at the highest risk for HIV have not been tested, usually because they do not realize that they are at risk. Others avoid testing because they are worried about the possibility of a positive test result. However, testing is encouraged because treatment for HIV is highly effective and learning about the infection can improve your chance of living longer and being healthier.

While getting tested is great, it should not be your method of prevention. Changing behaviors that put you at risk for HIV, open and honest communication, and mutual monogamy should be your goal.

Having the conversation about your sexual health and sex life may be difficult for yourself (and even your health care professional); however, no matter how uncomfortable the conversation may be, it is one that is necessary for your health and wellness. Besides, it could mean the difference between life and death!

Pearls of Wisdom: You are responsible for your sexual health! You must become the advocate to receive the necessary information, education and tools you need to keep yourself safer and to make healthier and informed decisions.

Importance of Knowing Your Reproductive System

IT IS EXTREMELY IMPORTANT TO become familiar with your reproductive system. After all, it is how we were created! It is an integral part of who we are! The reproductive system is just as important as all of the other systems in our bodies. They are all interrelated and work together to provide optimal health.

The more familiar you are with your body parts and how they function, the more you will be able to make healthier and informed decisions. You will also be able to educate and empower your loved ones with the knowledge, skills and tools they need to keep themselves safer. In addition, you will be able to experience more intimacy and sexual pleasure. In addition, you will be able to effectively communicate your beliefs, thoughts, wants, needs and desires to your Beloved.

Learning the proper terminology helps to remove language barriers and enables you to a have more informed conversation with your health care professional to get the care and treatment that you need. In addition, learning the proper terminology helps to add value to your body and when you value your body, you are less likely to place yourself at risk for STIs, unintended pregnancies and other emotional, mental, spiritual, social, legal, economical, chemical, energetical, political, institutional and physical consequences of sex.

Our bodies are a temple. We only get one, and there is no refund or exchange policy on our body, so we have to treat it with the utmost care and respect. If we do not take care of it, then who will? At the end of the day, you are responsible for your sexual health. It's time to break the cycle and reclaim your sexuality! Knowing and understanding the value of your reproductive system and body is the first step to enhancing your sexual pleasure.

I AM Sex: Part Three - I Am Ready for Pleasure

You Are Now Ready!

NOW THAT THE BLUEPRINT HAS been drawn and the foundation—understanding sexuality—has been laid, you are now ready to continue building on enhance my sexual pleasure! Let's define what sexual pleasure is—a beautifully choreographed dance of intimacy and intercourse between partners.

Before we go on, we must remember that sexual pleasure is so much more that intercourse. Sexual pleasure extends beyond the bedroom and transcends the all sexual dimensions of your life. Sexual pleasure can be a coupled experience or an intimate journey for one! It is a gift to yourself, or one that you share with others.

It is your right to experience sexual pleasure free of coercion, judgement, discrimination and violence! Experiencing sexual pleasure begins and ends with YOU! It is an acknowledgement and understanding of our own sexual needs and responsibilities. Ultimately, we are responsible for our own sexual pleasure, NOT our partners. We must be present, active and authentic in the experience. Only when we have acknowledged our pleasure can we begin to acknowledge and respond to the sexual needs and responsibilities of our partners.

Give yourself the permission!

Pearls of Wisdom: Sexual pleasure can be insatiable! The relentless pursuit of sexual pleasure can be harmful/dangerous. It can be just as gratifying as it can be deadly, so experience it wisely!

BENEDICTION

Silently we lay as we pray into each other's bodies
church has now begun
singing hymns and wailing praises
I testify it's mmmm so good
let the church say Amen
my God this man
reads my body like it's biblical scriptures
verse by verse
it's spiritual indeed
my body shouts hallelujah
as my energy comes alive
dancing and prancing
my hips sway into his come here motion
as I puddle into myself, he fills me
possessing me,
I-am possessing him
becoming sensations lost in the void of pleasure
I surrender my body to his rhythm
climbing higher and higher until I fall hard and fast
coming around him, I become undone
spiraling into orgasm, I now see myself in the light
yes! the doors are now open accepting his member
he thrusts hard in rhythmic motion bursting into fireworks
his head on my chest, arms under my back, legs wrapped around me
and in bliss we lay
passing the collection plate for a love offering is surely due
we bow our heads in reverence
and with all hearts, minds and bodies satisfied
let us now say....
Amen

Choreographing Your Sexual Pleasure

SEXUAL PLEASURE IS ALL ABOUT the choreography! Sexual choreography is a concept developed by Carole Rinkleib Ellison (although Ellison uses the concept in conjunction with Intimate-Based Sex Therapy for couples.) Intimate Based Sex Therapy is a holistic model that acknowledges an individual's mental, emotional, physical and spiritual factors in relationship to their self-esteem, intimacy, satisfaction and mutual pleasure. I have adapted the concept to fit within the framework of the sexual dimensions. Sexual choreography debunks the traditional belief of manufacturing orgasms and moves away from the linear model of sexual response originally presented by Masters and Johnson to and more comprehensive model of human sexual response, with considerations for all the sexual dimensions, such as the model that I presented earlier.

The sexual experience is aimed at enhancing sexual responsiveness and not only functionality; intercourse and orgasm are not required in order for an individual to experience sexual pleasure. Ellison states in her book that "success in a sexual interlude is defined not in terms of physiological function, but rather by creating a structure for erotic spontaneity that will enhance intimacy, facilitate sexual experience, mutual pleasure, and self-esteem" (Ellison, 2012, p. 144).

Sexual choreography is designed to help individuals and couples develop their sexual script and their rituals with the Dimensions of Sexuality according to their specific life situation. The couple is given specific activities that teach sexual negotiation, structure spontaneity, increase understanding and acceptance of variances in sexual styles, and focus attention during lovemaking and togetherness. The guiding assumption is that once an individual and/or couple have rewritten their sexual script, sexual pleasure will be enhanced due to an increase in intimacy and physical responsiveness.

INTIMACY VERSUS INTERCOURSE

Intimacy is a core component of sexual pleasure, thus enhancing the intimate connection helps to enhance sexual pleasure. We all desire to experience an intimate connection with our partner. We long for their tender kiss, soft and gentle caresses, intense eye contact and passionate sex—just like we see in the movies…right? Unfortunately, this unrealistic portrayal of intimacy actually limits our capacity for experiencing a true intimate connection with our partner. Creating such a connection requires willingness and work! So are you ready to take your relationship to the next level? By incorporating some of the ideas below into your relationship, you and your Beloved will be well on the way to creating the powerful and meaningful intimate connection that you so desire!

Eye Contact—The eyes are the gateway to the soul. Establishing eye contact helps to build an intimate connection between you and your partner. You may feel nervous and even vulnerable at first, but making eye contact during lovemaking lets your partner know that you are present and experiencing the moment with them. This helps to build trust, which ultimately leads to building and maintaining a more intimate relationship.

Touch—Kissing, massaging, stroking, and caressing all produce oxytocin, the bonding chemical. Touching each other throughout the day creates a feeling of closeness. Touching also helps to build desire for each other. Try touching each other without moving into intercourse. Building up the tension over the course of a few days can also lead to a deeper connection and more intense sexual encounter.

Breathing—Breathing together creates an instant connection between you and your partner. Synchronized breathing is a way to heighten pleasure, arousal and connection during lovemaking. When you breathe deeper, you bring more oxygen into the body, which heightens the intensity of arousal and orgasms. Sit in a "yab yum" position (face-to-face) and try alternating your breath as you breathe into each other's mouths; this exercise is very intimate and has been used in ancient traditions, such as tantric sex and Kama Sutra, as a way to share your soul.

Sexy Talk—Whispering sweet nothings into your lover's ear can instantly open their heart, not to mention sending blood rushing into their "ego." Try sending sexy emails, text messages and romantic reveries to your Beloved throughout the day. This not only builds anticipation, but it keeps your partner thinking about you all day, thus increasing the connection between you.

Do Something Extraordinary—Surprise your Beloved! Doing something extraordinary for your partner lets them know how much you care about them and that you're willing to go the extra mile to please them. You will be surprised at how much your partner will appreciate you for considering their needs and desires.

Allow Yourself to Be Vulnerable—It takes a lot to let down your guard, especially if you've been hurt before. Allowing yourself to be vulnerable by letting the walls around your heart melt gives your partner permission to penetrate you spiritually, intellectually, emotionally and physically. It also allows you to fully connect with your partner on all levels by experiencing the relationship in all its dimensions.

Cook Together—Creating a romantic dinner together offers opportunities for intimacy and closeness. Certain foods contain chemicals that are considered to have an aphrodisiac effect. Such foods include: ginger, curry, bananas, coconut, honey, oysters, saffron, soy, truffles, and artichokes. Additionally, chocolate is considered to create a lover's high because of the chemical phenylethylamine (PEA) that is responsible for the feelings of love and passion. Enjoy a sensual feast with your lover. Take time to feed each other while relishing in the aroma and flavors of the food.

Trying Something New—Be adventurous! Many couples get stuck with the bedroom blues when it comes to sex and intimacy. To break free of the monotony, try something new! Do something you have never done in bed, but have always wanted to. Take a class together at a sexy boutique, take a trip to a lingerie store, play sex games or introduce sex toys into your lovers' repertoire. Try watching an adult movie with your partner to learn some new moves.

Take a Dance Class—The argentine tango is sure to get the blood flowing between you and your Beloved! Dancing requires partnership and cooperation. It also increases the trust between you and your Beloved as you allow him/her to guide you effortlessly across the dance floor, holding you closely in their arms. In addition to being incredibly sexy, dancing is also a fun way to stay in shape and burn calories.

Set the Scene—Think of lovemaking as a theatrical piece. You need the right lighting, right mood, right props and costumes (or not). Set the scene for intimacy with sensual music, candles, soft fabrics, sexy toys, or even a different environment. Do not limit intimacy to the bedroom—you can also create a sensual experiences in the living room, kitchen or just about anywhere you can imagine! In all you do to set the scene, make sure you're set for an encore performance!

MAINTAINING THE HONEYMOON
Maintaining the intimacy can be particularly challenging, especially after the "honeymoon" period has faded into the background and life has begun to come into the forefront, overshadowing the relationship.

Remember the honeymoon phase—that initial romantic phase of love when you are so in love with your man or woman that you just cannot seem to get enough of each other. You're spending all your free time together, courting and dating, giggling, and the sex is frequent & fantastic! Everything is just right! You feel more alive with this person. However, one of the major drawbacks of this phase is that usually you're looking through rose-colored glasses and you fail to see the flaws, incompatibilities that may exist or the "little" things that you do not like about your Beloved which eventually become bigger things. Sometimes during the honeymoon phase, you are actually meeting the person's "representative," meaning that this person is doing everything right—cooking, sexing, cleaning the house—and all they can to get you. And once they got you, they hit you with the whom-doom! You are say to yourself, "Who in the hell are you?" Really good representatives can keep up the façade for years.

WHY DOES THE HONEYMOON PHASE COME TO AN END?

The reason why it seems like your once blissful relationship has taken a turn down hell's drive is due to the fact chemical response has dwindled off, causing the romantic stage to fade. You're no longer in that fantasy like state. Reality kicks in—you take off the rose-colored glasses and start to really see your Beloved for who they are, flaws and all. You realize that now you have to actually put the work into sustaining the relationship. In the beginning, everything is much easier because the chemicals secreted give you a positive attitude, increased energy, increased sexual desire and decreased need for sleep, which makes everything much easier. Now you have to work...and that is just too much for some people. Life changing events such as decline in health, or a dramatic change in work schedule may put unexpected strain on the relationship. All these factors combined begin to contribute a lack of intimacy and a significant decrease in sexual pleasure. So how does one keep begin to recreate the magic and keep the honeymoon going for years to come?

1. **Do not stop dating**. Although you are married or in a long-term committed relationship, you don't have to stop dating! Set aside time each month for you and your Beloved to go out on a date like you used to. It doesn't have to be an expensive date —a movie, dinner or nice long walk in the park with your sweetie, will do. Make date night a priority! Put the date on your calendar and be sure to keep it, even if it means rearranging your schedule or getting a sitter for the kids.

2. **Wear more lingerie**. Contrary to popular belief, husbands and boyfriends still enjoy and appreciate seeing their mates in sexy lingerie. Instead of frumpy old pajamas, try wearing a silky grown that grabs your body in all the right places, a girlie boy short set, or even his t-shirt to bed. Wearing matching bra and panties will not only turn him on, but it will make you feel good! Donning a nice piece of lingerie under your conservative business suit will make you feel powerful, feminine and sexy. At the end of the work day, surprise your lover with a strip tease, giving a whole new meaning to the phrase "working woman."

3. **Go out of your way and do something special**. Show your appreciation for your Beloved by treating him to something special every now and then. Pick up his favorite snack on the way home. Purchase a special item, a ticket to his favorite sporting event, or something that he normally would not purchase for himself. Men appreciate a woman that knows how and takes the time to show appreciation and respect for her man.

4. **Take care of yourself.** Keeping yourself up and maintaining your look is very important! Do not let yourself go after you get the man! It's not enough to look the part before the relationship. It's just as important (if not more so) to take care of yourself during the relationship. A man appreciates and respects a woman who takes care of herself. Taking care of yourself is also direct reflection of how you feel about yourself. While physical appearance is certainly not the only thing in a relationship, it is still a very

important aspect. Care enough about yourself to maintain your physical attributes by taking preventive health measures, eating right, exercising, drinking plenty of water and getting enough rest. Also, keeping your body clean is essential. Pay special attention to your genitalia—proper grooming is a must! Wear clothes that are flattering for your body type. Make-up is nice, but it isn't a must. However, if you chose to wear make-up, be sure to wear colors that compliment your complexion. Self-love is the most important type of love. If you cannot love and take care of yourself, then you cannot love and take care of anyone else, period!

5. **Keep a positive attitude**. "As a man thinketh, so is he." No one wants to be around a person who is negative and complains all the time. It is very unpleasant and can become very draining on one's spirit. Keeping a positive attitude is the key to happiness! We draw experiences to us based on our patterns of thought. By maintaining a positive outlook, you are more likely to create an atmosphere of peace. Additionally, you will be prepared to handle challenges that may come your way.

6. **Communicate, communicate, communicate!** Getting upset and shutting down is not the answer! Do not stop communicating your wants and needs, no matter how difficult it may be. Men are not mind readers. You cannot expect to have your wants and/or needs met without communicating them to your Beloved. Not communicating surely sets your Beloved up for failure, you for misery and eventually will become the demise of your relationship.

7. **Cook for your Beloved**. As the old adage says...the way to a man's heart is through his belly. Every man appreciates a good home-cooked meal every now and then. If cooking is not your forte, try taking a cooking class. Perhaps take a cooking class together to increase the intimacy and quality time between you and your Beloved. Most importantly, he will appreciate the thought and thank you for putting forth the effort on his behalf.

8. **Variety in the bedroom**. Every man loves a "bad girl!" Spice it up! Do not be afraid to try new things with your lover. The same old sex positions can become boring and monotonous. Try using a variety of sex positions. Pick up a book on Kama Sutra or Tantric Sex to increase intimacy, spirituality and sexuality. Also, incorporate the use of sex toys into your lovemaking. Make a day trip out of it! Visit a sex toy store together and purchase a fun new toy or how-to book, rent a sexy adult movie, go to a strip club and end your evening with a passionate night of lovemaking!

9. **Stroke his ego**. …literally and figuratively! Every man loves to be told how wonderful his is. It's important for him to feel wanted and needed by his woman. The phrase "gotta let a man be a man" is true. Find things that you love about your man and compliment him on it. Leave little love notes in his car, briefcase or on the bathroom mirror. Although we are strong, independent women, allow yourself to be vulnerable. It's ok every now and then to just become the "damsel in distress" and let him know that you need him. Also pay very special attention to your Beloved's manhood (i.e. penis). Make love to his penis with your mouth. Kiss, stroke and play with it on a regular basis. And no, ladies, it does not have to be a special occasion! As a matter of fact, out the blue is even better! Trust me; he will definitely appreciate you for it!

10. **Start things as you mean for them to go**. In other words, start your relationship off the way you intend to keep it going. We all start off new relationships by putting our best foot forward in an effort to attract, impress and keep the object of our desire. However, somewhere along the way those things we did in the beginning of the relationship somehow manage to fall by the wayside as we become settled. No one likes the old "bait and switch." If you start off the relationship by dressing a certain way or doing certain things, then it is those same things that you need to continue throughout the relationship. This helps

to provide a level of comfort and consistency, not to mention it shows your Beloved that you care enough to give him the best of you at all times.

11. **Don't lose yourself in him or her.** It is important to maintain a separate identity from your lover and your relationship. A sexy, confident person is a turn on for almost anyone; a person who knows who he or she is does not need someone else to define them. While it is important to have a mate, it is as equally important to maintain a sense of self and a certain level of independence within the relationship. A man needs to know that his woman has his back and that he can trust his woman to make certain decisions that will not be a deterrent to the relationship, her or his manhood. Never become predictable! Maintain your mystique—keep your partner guessing and you will keep him or her for life.

12. **Don't be overbearing, be supportive.** Do not become his mother! He already has one—he does not need another. One of your roles as loving mate is to be supportive and encouraging without being controlling. Men want a woman who is going to allow him to make his own decisions. Practice the art of listening. Men want to be heard more than they want advice. Learning the fine line between support and giving too much unwarranted and unwanted advice is important. Men need to learn on their own, without an "I told you so" from his woman. Even IF you already know, allow him the space to find out on his own. The only exception to this rule is if his decision will be detrimental to himself, you or the relationship. If you find this to be the case, then guide him ever so gently to the most appropriate solution.

Relationships are not always easy and they are certainly not fairytales. A loving relationship is a commitment through the good, bad and sometimes undesirable things that we learn about our partner. Relationships require a lot of active time to build and maintain their momentum. The key to longevity is the choices you make in the relationship! Although you may feel that the honeymoon phase has faded and you are stuck in a relationship rut, the great news is that you do not have to be! With love, commitment, dedication and a little work together, you and your Beloved can recapture the magic! Together, you both can remember all of the reasons why you fell in love and decided to build a life together. Let the process begin...view this new beginning with loving eyes, open hearts, and beauty as you embark on an intimate new journey of growth! The infinite honeymoon of happiness, health, love and sexual pleasure is well worth it!

JUST BUY THE LINGERIE!

Pearls of Wisdom: Buy the lingerie, but not just for the reasons you think!

So it is your anniversary, your Beloved's birthday, Valentine's Day or some other special occasion and you're shopping for the most fabulous piece of sexy lingerie you can find to help end your fantastic evening with a BIG Bang—no pun intended!

Stockings, stilettos, camis, babydolls, corsets and teddies help to provide an amazing erotic visual and go a long way in providing mental and visual stimulation for your partner, BUT the purchase of a quality piece of lingerie should be just as much, if not more, stimulating for you!

Victoria definitely knew and understood the power of the Secret! In addition to being aesthetically pleasing, the power of lingerie extends far beyond the mall and the bedroom. The principles of sensuality that go along with wearing lingerie help to enhance a woman in many other areas of her life: self-esteem, self-efficacy & confidence.

What we wear is often a direct reflection of who we are and how we feel about ourselves. The correlation between sensuality, sexuality, self-esteem and confidence and a fabulous piece of lingerie can definitely speak volumes about a woman. The type of lingerie a woman wears provides an outer expression of her inner sexuality—it says everything about you, your sexuality and how you project yourself. The more sexy the lingerie, the more likely she is to exude a confident attitude about herself and her body, and vice versa. This interconnectedness that is provided by wearing a beautiful piece of lingerie allows a woman to tap in to her feminine power to become the empowered women, feminine phenom, confident courtesan, sexy siren, vivacious vixen, beautiful bombshell or pin-up doll you so desire to be.

You do not have to wait until that "special" occasion or until your lover is around to adorn yourself in sexy lingerie. Every day is a special occasion in which you should celebrate yourself, and wearing lingerie should definitely be a part of that celebration! Stop lounging around the house all the time in baggy old sweats, oversized t-shirts, flannel pajamas and big fluffy robes. Try putting on a nice piece of lingerie to lounge around in the house. Try wearing it under your power business suit; you'd be surprised at how much more powerful you actually feel. Stop wearing granny panties and that ratty old bra and allow lingerie to be your sexy little secret that keeps you feel good and motivated throughout the day. You'll be amazed at how much more feminine, sexier, sensual and empowered you will feel, and this boost in your emotions will help to increase your overall feelings of self-love!

So the next time you are out lingerie shopping, keep in mind that your purchase is really for you. Take the time to select an haute couture piece that flatters your body type and speaks directly to you as if it were made specifically for you. Important things to consider when purchasing the perfect piece of lingerie include: 1) the type of lingerie i.e. corset, teddy, babydoll, 2) the color, 3) the material, 4) the functionality and 5) how does it make you feel? The perfect piece of lingerie should make you feel like the quintessential woman! Turn it into a fun shopping trip with your girlfriends, or even go on your own! If you want to be really naughty, invite your Beloved to accompany you and try on several pieces with the assistance of your Beloved and watch them melt with passion! Invite them into the fitting room for a little "retail therapy!"

Finally, once you've found the absolute perfect piece of lingerie and when you are ready for your big reveal (if your Beloved wasn't there when you purchased it) put it on and strut your stuff like the beautiful woman you are! Your Beloved will be so taken aback with your newfound confidence, sensuality & sexuality that they will ravish you in love...and they will be impressed with the lingerie you are wear too!

It's Spiritual

To taste your soul
so simply divine and if you don't mind
I'm ready....
let me
share in your delight til I feast
indeed
and in greed......indulge
for your sweetness is more than enough
to send me beyond myself only to find myself
as I melt into my emotions and cover you with me
I am spent and bent like elbows
for only heaven knows a feeling this actual and supernatural
so sweet
such that I see the God in you
staring back at me
and damn....it's spiritual
as we become
I exchange my love with yours
and we transcend beyond this space and time
yet only to find we were present the entire time
don't be afraid.....
its spiritual
as energy flows uniting yen with her yang
words cannot begin explain this
the mind cannot fathom an experience so surreal
how can I soar with an angels glow
don't you know.......
its spiritual
and so shall we dance
yes
let's dance sky Tantra to our beating hearts become one in rhythmic meter

my God my soul has found her mate
and yes…..
it's spiritual
it's emotional, it's sexual, it's effectual,
it's Love!
yes, it's Love!
yes, my God it's…..Love

Intimacy Beyond Intercourse

TANTRA

Tantra is one of the oldest known arts of sacred sexuality practiced today. Although Tantra has long been practiced in many eastern cultures, it is just beginning to flourish in the United States. Born in India more than 6,000 years ago, Tantra emerged as a rebellion against organized religion, which held that sexuality should be rejected in order to reach enlightenment. Tantra challenged the acetic beliefs of that time, purporting that sexuality was a doorway to the divine, and that earthly pleasures, such as eating, dancing and creative expression were sacred acts.

The essence of Tantra lies in the ability to transform sexual energy into a spiritual journey to nirvana, bridging the gap between spirituality and sexuality thus awakening to full enlightenment and awareness. Tantra is a "practical" spiritual path that is practiced in sacredness. Since Tantra is practiced as a spiritual ritual, as with all forms of spiritual worship, there is an acknowledging and honoring of a divine presence or being. In the case of Tantra, this is reflected by acknowledging and honoring the divine presence of God in your partner and each other throughout the realm of the senses.

From the beginning, Tantric teachings passed from one generation to the next in the unwritten form of the rituals themselves, then later through writings known simply as "Tantras." The Tantras were written in Sanskrit and are composed of dialogues between the Hindu god Shiva and the Hindu goddess Shakti. A Sanskrit (ancient Hindu) word,

Tantra means to expand, join or weave Yin (female) and Yang (male) energy between lovers. This joining of the polarities of male (represented by the Hindu god, Shiva), and female (embodied by the Hindu goddess, Shakti), incorporates them into a harmonious unit of one in which they reach the essence of their core identity through a variety of rituals in the mental, emotional, spiritual and sexual dimensions of wellness.

The weaving of the Tantric energy is based on the balance of the chakras (energy wheels). According to Tantric beliefs, there are seven chakras which align the center of the body. When in proper balance, the chakras allow us to understand the relationship between our highest consciousness and physical being. Tantra focuses specifically on using the chakras to direct Kundalini (sexual) energy between Yin & Yang within the six essential elements of Tantra: breath, movement, muscle lock, sound, intention and attention. When a deep interconnection is established throughout all of the six essential elements, the perceived space between yin and yang becomes filled with the light of Spirit. This spiritual presence activates energy between the two, joining them as one.

TANTRIC SEX VERSUS WESTERNIZED SEX

Tantra is different from western ideas about sex. In the West, we sometimes view sex as a source of recreation rather than a means of transformation. The goal may be to reach orgasm rather than to pleasure our lover or to connect with him or her more fully. Another key distinction between westernized views of sex and tantric sex is that the western sexual script has a clear beginning (sexual excitement), middle (penetration), and end (orgasm). Sex is seen as goal-oriented, with orgasm being the end result and any adaptation from this script being perceived as wrong.

Tantric sex is not result- or goal-oriented, but rather, timeless and unstructured. In Tantric sex, the point of sex is not orgasm—the point is to experience the sensations and pleasures associated with intimate connection with a partner. There is no clear cut beginning, middle, or end. Most of the exercises related to Tantric sex involve slowing things down, trying not to focus on our external body, or orgasm, or anything outside of the experience of the moment. Without a focus on orgasm, sex becomes more about exchanging pleasures, awakening the senses and allowing couples to communicate on deep physical and emotional levels. During this time, lovers are able to establish an intimate connection that can be maintained and heightened as they transition into the sexual dimension.

Another major difference between the westernized way of sex and Tantric sex is the emphasis of breathing and slowing down sexual behavior compared to the hectic, orgasm-focused westernized approach. In the art of Tantra, there are a variety of individual and partnered activities that are designed to focus on breathing and meditation. The activities and exercises help to bring attention, focus and intention into the moment. In addition, breathing directs energy, frees emotions, and increases stamina and orgasmic intensity as oxygen is dispersed throughout the muscles and bloodstream.

Tantra can be a very breathtaking (literally & figuratively) journey especially when practiced with a partner who is open to transcending into a spiritual journey while experiencing sexual ecstasy. The benefits to Tantric sex are endless. Some benefits of Tantra include the ability to delay orgasm, the ability to heal past emotional wounds, deepening a connection to your partner, rejuvenation of health, and the ability to experience ecstatic sexual states. Practicing Tantra will increase intimacy, energy of attraction, communication, and spirituality, ultimately enhancing the richness of the relationship. Through its rituals, Tantra teaches ways to carry this intense focus of concentration into all areas of life. The rituals make it possible to enjoy not only sex, but increase happiness in all other dimensions in one's life.

Tantric sex extends far beyond the bedroom by helping partners open fully to each other in trust and love through all facets of their relationship and creating a space for spiritual growth and personal awareness. As you learn to open yourself to the path of love, you naturally open to others around you. You begin to understand that surrender does not mean submission or loss of self, but rather a loving expansion to something that is much greater than you are. The practice of Tantric sex shows us how to reclaim the sexual intimacy that is our inherent birthright. Through this most ancient of art, we discover new joys of the erotic pleasure and expand our moments of sexual ecstasy into a lifetime of happiness and bliss. The real essence of Tantra cannot be captured in oral or in written words. To truly understand Tantra, you have to experience it!

The First Time We Made Love

Hearts beating simultaneously
breathing as one
for this is no ordinary love
picture this
body's intertwine
glistening
trembling helplessly
fluids flowing abundantly
uninhibited
so satisfying
liquid voices fill the air
echoing from beyond
soulful moans
sighs of release
we lay enrapt in the memory
captured by this very moment
for our eyes don't lie
telling a story of pleasure undefiled
smiles reveal our delight
the first time we made love
was an unforgettable Saturday morning

Sexual Intercourse

"Earth shattering, mind-blowing, sheet-biting sex doesn't just happen like in the movies! Most people's sex life won't ever reach its full potential because they're just not willing to step outside box...they have become too comfortable with the old familiar things, or they're just not willing to put in the work!"

—Dr. TaMara

Are You Ready for Sex?

The expression of your sexual self through intercourse is an amazing gift that you give only to someone that you feel is worth receiving one of your most valued possession, because once you give yourself to someone, you cannot take it back! In addition, once you give yourself to someone sexually, you form a lasting emotional, mental, spiritual, social, chemical, energetical, physical and sometimes a legal and economical bond!

Sexual intercourse can also provide a way to express intimate intentions, love and pleasure; as well as learn about yourself and the ways in which you communicate sexually with other people. Sex is also deeply personal. So personal that you actually open yourself literally, figuratively and physically to allow someone into your womanhood, since you are the receiving partner. This intense experience can result in feelings of overwhelming vulnerability which can leave you with an array of feelings to sort though. This is why it is extremely important that you are very conscious of who you chose to share yourself with. Because as I mentioned before, once you give yourself away.....you can NOT take it back.

Do not take the decision to have sex lightly! Your sexual expression is uniquely and authentically yours, and only you can decide when you're ready to have sex.

"Although the physical act of sex or intercourse is definitely an important component to our sexuality and relationships, we spend far too much time only focusing on that component. As a result, we become out of balance in the other dimensions of our sexuality. When we are out of balance, our entire life begins to suffer." -Dr. TaMara

POSITIONS AND TECHNIQUES ARE ONLY PART OF THE WHOLE OF SEXUALITY

We spend so much time focusing on finding the most stimulating positions and perfecting technique that we often miss the experience of intercourse. We are so busy concentrating on the ultimate *goal* of orgasm that we fail to be present for ourselves and/or our partners. Goal-oriented intercourse leaves us, (and sometimes our partners) feeling frustrated and dissatisfied both emotionally and physically. This dissatisfaction can lead to complications in relationships, feelings of worthlessness, body image issues, sexual dysfunctions, resentment, bitterness and so much more.

The goal of sexual activity for women is not necessarily orgasm, but rather personal satisfaction, which can manifest as physical satisfaction (orgasm) and/or emotional satisfaction (a feeling of intimacy and connection with a partner). When we enter into the experience in terms of pleasure versus goal, we are better able to relax, be present and feel the pleasure.

A great sex life is all about growing into a mutually sexually satisfying relationship that grows and flourishes over time and involves mutual submission, selflessness, pleasure, intimacy, bonding, communication and of course intercourse; however, there is certainly space for learning about sexual positions and techniques and practicing them as part of our sexual expression of physical intimacy with our Beloved.

SEXUAL POSITIONS

I am not going to spend a lot of time talking about sexual positions. I know this may be a disappointment to some, because after all, this is a book about sex, right? The reason behind this decision is because there are so many great books out there already that are focused on sexual position and technique. While position and technique are definitely significant to sexual pleasure, *I AM Sex* offers a more holistic and comprehensive view that is more focused on the overall aspect of sexuality.

Additionally, I choose not to spend a lot of time on sexual positions and technique because it is truly an individual and/or couple preference. What worked for one person and one relationship may not necessarily work for another person or another relationship. So in terms of what the best position and/or techniques are, I would say the one that works best for you and your Beloved! This is why sexual communication and willingness to explore with your partner is so important! With that being said, I encourage you to talk with your partner about what turns you on, and what makes you feel good. Tell him or her what your hot spots are.

Homework: For the next month, your assignment is to go to a book store, preferably with your Beloved, and pick up a book of sexual positions. Go home and explore the book together. Pick out some of your favorite positions and get busy! If the first few positions do not move you, then continue to try different positions until you find the one that makes you and your Beloved's bodies move in rhythmic motion/sync like a perfect, sexually-charged choreographed routine!

Below are some helpful hints that may allow you experience more pleasure during sexual intercourse:

Pillows Work Wonders. You know, those decorative pillows can be used for more than making the bed look pretty! They can also be used to help alleviate pain and make you feel great during sex. Pillows can help by reducing the amount of sling action and tension. They can also help align the body. There are companies that make specialized pillows specifically for sex. They are great—however, they tend to be a bit expensive.

Synchronize Your Body. Become a slave to the rhythm! Keep your body in sync with your partner. Aligning your bodies during sex will help to make penetration much easier. Flowing together with the same rhythmic motion will not only minimize pain, but also help to synchronize movements and breathing which will help increase intimacy. Additionally, it increases your partner's chances of hitting all the right spots!

Increase Body Awareness. Become intimately acquainted with your body movements on a daily basis. Learn what movements result in pleasure and pain—this type of awareness will help you identify movements that may result in pleasure and pain during sex. Additionally, it helps you to be present and more in tune with intercourse, resulting in mind-blowing orgasms.

Avoid the Jerk. If you have lower back pain, avoid sexual positions that involve a lot of thrusting. Also, avoid sudden jerking movements—instead transition gently from one position to the next. Keeping your neck and back aligned will also help to reduce pain. Abrupt moves always ruin the mood and the orgasm.

Be Aware of the Legs. Lifting your legs can be a real strain, especially if you already have lower back problems or if your leg muscles are not flexible. Over-extending the legs during sex can also lead to fatigue and cramping. To minimize the aching on the legs, use pillows to prop up your legs or positions that allow you to use your partners body for support. Relax those legs!

Changing It Up. Stop having sex in the same old way! Experiment with different positions and techniques to see what works for both of you. It can be a challenge at first, but it helps to break the monotony, adds creativity and helps to alleviate pain. Remember, variety is the spice of life!

Communicate. Great sex doesn't just happen like it does in the movies. While it may be challenging to communicate your sexual desires to your Beloved, it is absolutely necessary! Oftentimes, we set our relationships up for failure because we don't to talk to our partners. We just "expect" them to somehow know everything about us. Don't expect your Beloved to be a mind reader! You have to communicate with each other about what turns you on and off because what worked with one partner may or may not necessarily do it for the current partner. Be very specific about what you need. Rather than criticizing your Beloved about the things that you don't like, instead tell them what feels good and what you want more of. You can also take their hands and gently guide them to your "*hot spots.*"

Knowing is half the battle! Don't assume or pretend to know what your partner needs. When in doubt ask questions—preferably before sex and not during, because that can certainly spoil the mood! Try not to become offended when your Beloved tells you his or her desires. It's not a slam against you; but rather, a suggestion on how to increase their pleasure. After all, your focus is to have the best sex possible, right? Be open to loving suggestions from your partner!

Sharing your sexual desires will not only enhance your relationship in and out of the bedroom, but it can also create an unparalleled level of intimacy between you and your Beloved. Your willingness to explore sexual desires together can take you into exciting new territory far away from your old, boring sex script!

Don't forget the foreplay. Sometimes a quickie is great, but don't forget the foreplay! Women need foreplay to help get their natural juices flowing. In addition, foreplay helps to lengthen the vagina so that she is able to welcome your manhood into her sanctuary. Now I know you're probably thinking that foreplay takes way too long. Well, it's time for you to think outside the box! Foreplay can begin long before the bedroom romp-a-rama session. Build excitement and anticipation throughout the day so that by the time you're ready to do the horizontal mambo, she's literally dripping wet for you! Ladies don't be too selfish—men like fore-play too! Leave his favorite pair of your sexy undies in his pocket so he can find it later! Greet him at the door in a Dominatrix outfit ready to subdue him with your feminine prowess or get him all cleaned up and prepared for sex wearing a sexy French maid outfit!

Add variety. Variety is the spice of life! It may be cliché, but yet so true! Any great chef knows that it's the variety of seasonings, textures and flavors that makes the dining experience great. The same thing is true for sex! It's easy to get stuck in the same old boring sex rut, but now it's time for you to spice things up a bit! Positively persuade your partner into trying something new. Make an adventure out of it by planning a fun day trip. Start your blood flowing by getting a couples' massage, get up close and personal during a boudoir photo shoot, visit an adult novelty and purchase a fun new sex toy or rent a sexy adult movie, and end your evening with a passionate night of lovemaking. Can't think of any new positions? Pick up a book on Kama Sutra or Tantric Sex to help increase your intimate, emotional and spiritual connection.

Practice Makes Perfect. If at first you don't succeed then try, try again! To be the best at anything, you must learn all the tricks of the trade… pun intended! You must hone your skills and perfect your craft to get it right. All the great athletes, entertainers and entrepreneurs did not become the greatest overnight, nor did they experience success without discipline, study and practice. If you want to perform better sexually, it's going to take some work and maybe even learning some new things. To further our careers and to cultivate our growth, we attend professional developments classes to enhance our skills. Because our bodies, lives and sex will change overtime, we need to be continuous learners. So grab your lube, toys, imagination and partner, because school is in session!

Let Go! Stop concentrating so much and allow your body to relax. Holding your body so tightly during sex constricts your blood. Additionally, when we are tense, our muscles tighten up causing pain. Let go and allow the energy to flow through your body to increase your pleasure and orgasmic intensity.

Speaking of the BIG "O"

PEARLS OF WISDOM: PEOPLE WHO experience orgasms often look like they are in pain. In fact, two of the brain regions that are activated by pain are also activated during orgasm, perhaps accounting for the curious similarity of facial expressions. Scientists are unsure how the brain distinguishes between pain and pleasure.

Orgasm is a physical, emotional, mental and spiritual response experienced at the height of sexual activity. Orgasm is also a biological release of chemicals and tension, followed by pleasurable involuntary muscle contractions.

There's a lot of pressure on women regarding orgasms! Many articles, books, etc. can make a women feel inadequate. But the interesting thing is that woman are experiencing orgasm but because they did not receive proper sexuality educations, not in tune with their body or are often not informed on the various types of orgasms that she can experience, in her mind….she has not.

There are several types of orgasms a woman can experience: clitoral, vaginal, A-Spot G-spot, anal, full body, blended and multiple! I know you are probably thinking, "wait...I can have all those different types of orgasms?" The answer is yes! The good news is that since you know, you can now look forward to experiencing mélange of orgasms

CLITORAL ORGASM

The clitoris is the pleasure spot specially designed for women. It is the most sensitive area on the female body, being one of the most nerve rich—over 8,000. The vast majority of women experience clitoral orgasm through direct stimulation or indirect stimulation of the internal structure of the clitoris. Intensely pleasurable feelings start within the clitoris and send waves of pleasure throughout the body.

VAGINAL ORGASM

A vaginal orgasm begins deep in the vagina near the cervix and either stays focused in the pelvic and lower stomach areas. In fact, many women do not even realize that are experiencing a vaginal orgasm because it begins so deep inside of the vagina. A vaginal orgasm may or may not happen in unison with a clitoral orgasm. During a vaginal orgasm, the uterus and pelvic muscles contract. The contractions are so strong that they can actually push anything that is inside of the vagina out, like a penis or sex toy. A vaginal orgasm takes longer to achieve. Continuous rhythmic thrusting is often the best way to bring a woman to a vaginal orgasm.

A-SPOT ORGASM (THE ANTERIOR FORNIX ORGASM)

The A-Spot is located about 4-5inches deep on the front wall of the vagina. An A-Spot orgasm is achieved by stimulating this small patch of sensitive tissue that is located near the cervix. When stimulated, the A-Spot can lead to rapid vaginal lubrication and arousal.

Also referred to as the *Epicentre*, this is a patch of sensitive tissue at the inner end of the vaginal tube between the cervix and the bladder, described technically as the 'female degenerated prostate.' (In other words, it is the female equivalent of the male prostate, just as the clitoris is the female equivalent of the male penis.) Direct stimulation of this spot can produce violent orgasmic contractions. Unlike the clitoris, it does not suffer from post-orgasmic over-sensitivity.

G-Spot

The G-Spot is located about 2-3 inches inside the vagina on the front wall. The G-Spot is about the size of a nickel and the texture of the G-spot is much more spongy and coarse than the rest of the vagina. During sexual arousal, the tissue surrounding the urethra becomes engorged with blood and the Para-urethral/Skenes glands produce and fill with fluid. The fullness of the gland stimulates the feeling of needed to urinate. This is partly because of the pressure of the fluids surrounding the glands of the urethra. Additionally, G-Spot orgasms are responsible for female ejaculation. It may be difficult for a woman to locate her G-Spot; however, it becomes much easier to find after she has had one orgasm.

Anal Orgasm

The anus is an erogenous zone full of sensitive nerves. Additionally, the sphincter muscle creates intense sensations when it contracts. However, because the anus does not lubricate itself naturally, lots of lubrication—water-based or silicone-based—must be used during any anal play. There are several ways you can reach anal orgasm: manual stimulation; using a sex toy such as a vibrator, dildo, butt plug or anal beads; oral-anal sex; or penile penetration.

Cervical Orgasm

The cervix is the entrance to the womb, the uterus. A woman's cervix is related to her feminine core, her sense of self, her heart, her creativity, and to her entire being. According to the Tantric tradition, a cervical orgasm is probably the most profound, meaningful orgasm a woman can experience. A cervical orgasm is characterized by contractions of the deep vaginal muscles and uterus. The sensation of cervical stimulation and orgasm feels different from clitoral stimulation, because they are responding to two different nerve-systems. A cervical orgasm will feel deeper, more intense and is accompanied by strong emotions, love, oneness with self, partner and god, ecstasy and transcendence, tears, crying and a feeling of deep satisfaction on all levels.

BLENDED ORGASM

A blend orgasm is one of the most powerful orgasms a woman can experience. It offers a woman the best of both worlds. A blended orgasm is a potent combination of two or more types of orgasms occurring at the same time.

MULTIPLE ORGASMS

Contrary to popular belief, multiple orgasms do exist, and they are entirely possible to achieve if there is little to no interruption in arousal or stimulation. Multiple orgasms come in quick succession, one after the other, usually with mere seconds to minutes between them. The challenge with multiple orgasms is that due to the heighten sensitivity, continued orgasm may become uncomfortable if stimulation is continued. There are two types of multiple orgasms: sequential and serial. Sequential orgasms are orgasms that occur after one another with a few minutes in between. Additional stimulation is often required to get from one to the next, but there is no limit to how many you might have during one encounter. Serial orgasms are one orgasm experienced immediately after the next (and the next and the next.)

FULL BODY/EXPANDED ORGASM

A full body/expand orgasm is associated with Tantra. It can be described as a true "floating-on-cloud-nine, out of body" experience. A full body/ expanded orgasm is the experience of feeling your whole body vibrating with orgasmic intensity and contractions that last from a few minutes to many hours. These contractions and energetic sensations pulsate all over the body, especially in the abdomen, inner thighs, hands, feet, and genitals bringing about deep emotional release and rejuvenation, profound spiritual experiences, and a keen awareness not normally perceived in other types of orgasms. A full body/expanded orgasm uses the body, mind, emotion, spirit and sexual energy to create your purpose.

When it comes to orgasms, it is important to note that orgasms vary in intensity, and women vary in the frequency of their orgasms and the amount of stimulation necessary to trigger an orgasm and even what type of orgasm she experiences. Additionally, orgasms are affected by cognitive, psychological, environmental and pharmacological variables.

Stop comparing your orgasmic experience to that of your girlfriends. No two orgasms are alike, not even your own. Because the genitals are connected to several different pairs of nerves, stimulating different combinations of nerves produces different sensations. The important thing is to know your body and tune into your sexual response. The more in tune you are, the more likely you will be able to experience an orgasm.

Pearls of Wisdom: Orgasms get better with age. As women mature and become more sexually empowered, they have more confidence during sex and therefore are able to experience more pleasure.

Pearls of Wisdom: Women can delay orgasm through a variety of ways. For example, in some practices of Hinduism—such as Tantra, which emphasizes sexual intercourse for religious purposes—techniques allow some individuals to control ejaculation and orgasm.

EXPERIENCING THE ULTIMATE ORGASM

The quest to experience the ultimate orgasm is a challenge that many women will face throughout their lives. The mysteries of the female orgasm, however, lies not so much in what physiological effects they cause, but rather how to experience more and better orgasms. The more a woman knows about her own body, how it changes throughout the various stages of the Human Sexual Response Cycle, the different types of orgasms and orgasm techniques, increases the likelihood of having orgasms alone and/or with your partner. Below are some additional suggestions to enhance your orgasmic pleasure.

* First, you may want to consult with your physician to rule out any medical condition that may be contributing to your inability to experience an orgasm.

* Mind play. Keep in mind that sex begins in the brain. Any emotional or mental blocks during foreplay and/or intercourse will make it difficult to experience an orgasm.

* Know your body. Always be aware of how you enjoy being touched sexually. You must communicate this openly and honestly with your partner. Share with him how you liked to be touched. Lovingly teach him and guide his hands all over your body.

* Seduction is the key! Women need to be engaged in a lot of foreplay prior to intercourse. Set the mood—don't just jump right into it. Take your time and allow your intensity to build, as this will help to increase the intensity of your orgasm.

* Try different positions. This allows for different types of stimulation of the vagina, G-spot, A-Spot and clitoris.

* Try using sex toys to bring yourself to orgasm. There are a variety of sex toys on the market designed for specific usage. You may consider a clitoral vibrator or a g-spot vibrator to start you on your journey.

* Take your time—don't rush to orgasm. Enjoy the full sexual experience, and slowly build up to your orgasm. If you can hold out, try to "edge"—control yourself just shy of the actual orgasm for as long as possible. The result of edging can be an extremely intense orgasm that will be accompanied with stronger contractions and a longer lasting climax.

* Strengthen your PC muscles. Pubococcygeal muscles are a big part of the female orgasm. Try exercising your muscles using Ben Wa Balls, vaginal or Kegel Exercisers. The stronger the PC, muscle the more intense the orgasm.
* Understand the Human Sexual Response Cycle. Having an understanding of how your body responds during each phase of the human sexual response cycle will help to increase your chances of experiencing an orgasm.
* Relax into pleasure. Stop having goal-oriented sex. Don't focus so much on the goal, but rather experiencing the sensuality and pleasure of your sex play.

Always remember that the most immediate route to orgasm is direct stimulation of the clitoris, as it is the only organ in the female body whose sole purpose is to provide pleasure! Just like with anything else, practice makes perfect! Take your time and be gentle and loving with yourself! Good things "come" to those who wait!

FROM HIS TONGUE TO MINES

From inside I feel the pleasures of your tongue
releasing passion held captive within
I moan
squirming ever so gently back and forth
I make love to your smile
wrapping your hands around my waist
pulling me closer to your face
I mount your shoulders in pure ecstasy
for it has got to be a sin to feel this good
I drip with desire
let your fingers swim in my natural delight
as you continue to take me into your mouth, you taste me
as you continue to make me
tingle to vibration, tremble with intensity
I cum and cum and cum
now kiss me
and let me taste myself
for nothing else
could be this sweet

Communicating Your Sexual Desires?

Q. How do I tell my partner that I want more of the same (sexually) without bruising his ego?

A. Talk to your partner about the great times you've already had in bed. Be very specific about what you need. Rather than criticizing your partner about the things you don't like, say exactly what you love and tell him you want more of it. You can also take his hands and gently guide them to your "hot spots." As you guide his hands, be sure to moan and groan to indicate that you are turned on and enjoying it. These two techniques will help to ensure that your partner is giving you what you want. Boosting his confidence because he knows he's pleasing you will equal mind-blowing orgasms for both of you!

In order to experience unparalleled levels of intimacy and optimal pleasure, it is important that we learn to communicate our sexual desires. Sharing your sexual desires can not only empower you with newfound confidence both in and out of the bedroom, your willingness to explore your sexual desires together can take you into exciting new territory far away from your old, boring sex script.

COMMUNICATION BUILDS INTIMACY

Intimacy is so much more than hot, steamy sex! It extends far and beyond the confines of the bedroom or wherever you chose to have sex! Intimacy is an essential building block of relationships. It's the glue that binds two individuals together. It's a choice to expose the very depths of your mind, body, spirit and soul! Of course intimacy includes: kissing, holding hands, eye contact, doing things together like taking a class, sharing past and present experiences, exposing our vulnerability and building emotional connections by communicating our fears, dreams, wants, needs, desires, etc.

COMMUNICATION ENHANCES SEXUAL PLEASURE

When you learn to communicate your sexual desires, it takes the sexual experience to a whole new level because now you are actively engaged in the process. You're an involved participant, not just lying there hoping that your partner pleases you (which, by the way, is not their responsibility). We must not only show up, but be present in every experience in our lives in order to reap the total benefits. Sexual activity is no different. At the end of the day, your partner is going to make sure that they are satisfied, so why shouldn't you?

COMMUNICATION EMPOWERS YOU TO TAKE
CONTROL OF SEXUAL EXPERIENCES

When you communicate your sexual desires, not only does it enhance your pleasure, but it puts you in control of your experience. This is important because sometimes when we look for other people to satisfy us or handle things, we are often times left unfulfilled with the short end of the stick. Who is to blame? We are. We have to be willing to speak up and advocate for our pleasure. We have to be courageous and bold enough to tell our partners, (in a loving way, of course) what's working and what's not working for us. We have to be able to say, "I love when you do this. It feels so good to me and turns me on. I need more of this (and not so much of that) because this gets me off every time." As long as you say things in a loving manner, you're not bruising their ego by telling them what they've done wrong or what you don't like, because who wants to hear that, right? Instead, stroke their ego and building them up by telling them all that they are doing that makes you feel good. Please believe when you say it to them that way, you will get what you want every time because at the end of the day, even though it's not their sole responsibility, our partners really want to please us!

STOP FAKING ORGASMS!

Q. *Am I wrong for faking an orgasm when I am having sex with my boyfriend? I just want it to be over because he is just not pleasing me.*

A. *Faking an orgasm definitely sends the wrong message to your boyfriend. He will think that he's pleasing you, when in fact he's not. Instead of faking it, have a conversation with him about your likes and dislikes. "Teach" him what really turns YOU on. Consider incorporating some lover's games" into the mix so that it becomes something fun and exciting for the both of you. Also, explore different positions, stimulations, toys, etc. This conversation should take place prior to (and not during) sex. Be sure to be as loving as possible so that you don't bruise his ego. The conversation should also take place in a neutral location, not the bedroom. Remember, it is not necessarily your boyfriend's responsibility to give you an orgasm. You are responsible for your own pleasure, so you must be an active participant too!*

Now I know at some point, we all have faked an orgasm! I know I'm not the only one. We laid there moaning and groaning, and even making a face or two while our Beloved partners thought they were putting in work and pleasing us, when actually they were not. We left the experience feeling more frustrated and sometimes even hornier than before. Whose fault is that? Ours…yup ours!

When we don't communicate, it sends the wrong message to our partners. When we don't talk with our partners and tell then exactly how we feel about our sexual experiences, we do them and ourselves a disservice. It is a disservice to them because they think that they may be pleasing us when in fact they are not. It is a disservice to us because we don't receive the most pleasure that we can from our sexual experience. It's important to always remember that we are responsible for our sexual health and pleasure—that is why it is extremely important that we learn how to communicate our wants, needs and desires.

SO HOW DO I TALK TO MY BELOVED ABOUT MY SEXUAL DESIRES?

Talking with your Beloved about your sexual desires must be handled in a very non-threatening, non-judgmental manner. Timing is also important. Creating a safe space that is conducive to sharing will also help the discussion.

Telling your partner that you want to try something new sexually can be stressful no matter how fantastic your relationship is. Talking about your sexual desire will be easier if you already have great communication and an openness to talk about sex. However if you normally don't talk about sex in your relationship, your sudden interest to do so may incite questions from your partner. Your Beloved may wonder where this sudden desire is coming from or even if you've had sexual secrets all along. If this is the case, allow your partner the time and space to ask questions that s/he may have as this may be an opportunity to open up and begin to explore your sex lives together.

Keep in mind that when you are introducing your sexual desires, especially new ones, to your Beloved; you may be met with excitement, hesitation, interest, reluctance and even a flat out refusal to engage in conversation and/or entertain the sexual desire. If you are met with a less than enthusiastic response, don't push the issue, as it will only make things worse. Remember it is your partner's right to process their feelings regarding your sexual revelation.

Before you come clean and confess your innermost sexual desire to your partner, think about how you can bring the subject up in a way that feels safe and non-threatening to your partner. Think about things you can say to encourage your partner to hear you out, and ask them to delay judgment and responses until you finish explaining the sexual desire and why it is important to you.

Now, here are some additional helpful tips to introducing new sexual desires into your relationship:

* Remember to remind your Beloved how much you love them. Nothing can replace the bond shared between a woman and a man. Just because you'd like to introduce a new desire doesn't mean that they weren't pleasing you before—it just simply means that you would like to take the sex play to another level of pleasure by enhancing what you're already doing.

* Use books, pictures, videos, etc. to help explain your sexual desire. Some people are visual. Showing them exactly what you mean can help to lovingly persuade them. People fear the unknown or what they do not understand. By using a visual aid, it can help to relax their fears because they can actually see what you're talking about which can actually help to peak their curiosity and excitement and encourage them to try it.

* Do not bring up new sexual desires during the midst of your sex play, as this can result in disaster. Nothing can spoil the mood more than telling your partner what you don't like while they believe that they are pleasing you. Not only will it ruin the mood and cause them to stop, but it may also result in hurt feelings and some alone time for you.

* Have the conversation in a neutral and relaxed environment. Don't have this conversation in the bedroom. The bedroom is supposed to be a sanctuary, a place of peace, relaxation and sleep, not deep conversations. Consider having the conversation over a nice dinner or walk in the park, some place that is

neutral and comfortable for both. The movies, sporting event or any other loud event that can be distracting or does not allow of conversation is not a good place.

* Watch a movie together or read a scene from an erotic novel that illustrates your desire and use it as a starting point for a discussion. This is an easy way to start the discussion and a great way to learn about what pleases your Beloved in an informal way.

* Reassure them that you wouldn't bring up the idea unless you felt safe to share your deepest desires with them. Remember, relationships are supposed to be about trust, sharing and building an intimate bond. You should be able to share your desires with your partner without feeling anything other than loved and supported.

* Positively persuade your partner by telling them how much fun the two of you can have exploring & trying something new. We all like new things. The only thing better than new things is getting something else new. Think of this as your own personal scavenger hunt that the two of you can go on, with the prize being the ultimate orgasm!

* Explain how your sexual desire will benefit the relationship by increasing intimacy between you two. Whenever we are doing something that we truly enjoy, dopamine pumps this "feel good" sensation throughout our body. When released, it produces feelings of pleasure and satisfaction. Now couple that with oxytocin, affectionately labeled "the bonding hormone," which is also released during sexual activity, producing feelings of trust, emotional intimacy, relaxation, attachment and contentment between people. Dopamine calms the spirit and lifts moods, reducing fear and anxiety and allowing a feeling of safety in the arms of your Beloved.

* Most importantly, communicate your feelings in a loving manner. Be supportive and not overbearing. Try not to place blame or pressure on your partner as this will only create more stress and tension ultimately making the situation worse. Be loving

and be patient. Remember, things did not get this way overnight, therefore you cannot expect change overnight. It's a process that is well worth the journey!

* Anytime we over-indulge in substances, prescription, legal or illegal, our mental state becomes altered. When we are not in our sober frame of mind, our judgment may lapse and our inhibitions go out the door. We tend to make decisions that we would not normally make if we were not under the influence. (say hurtful things to your Beloved, have unprotected sex or even have sex with someone we normally would not). In addition, our hormones are more active after a night of drinking, drugging and partying; therefore, we are more likely to give in to the animalistic urge to have sex.

Sexperiment with Your Sexual Script!

No LONGER IS SEX TABOO, nor does it carry all the societal stigma that it once used to. From television shows to movies, radio and video, people are increasingly becoming more in-tune with their sexuality and opening up about their sexual desires. Bored with "traditional" sex scripts and roles, people are deciding to step outside the boundaries of "regular" sex and opting for something a little more exciting and risqué. Tapping into your sexuality and exploring your sexual desires can be a very pleasurable and invigorating experience. So if you're ready to turn it up a notch and unleash the sexual beast within, here are some ways to "sexperiment" to help keep your sex life fresh and interesting!

Sexual Preferences. Whether you consider yourself to be bisexual, heteroflexible, heterocurious, questioning, or just plain ole curious, there is fluidity in sexuality. According to Alfred Kinsey, the famous sex researcher, very few of us lie at polar opposites on the sexual continuum from heterosexual to homosexual, but somewhere in between. Kinsey also goes on to suggest that based on a variety of activities, individuals may move back and forth on the continuum. So based on that theory, there is a natural inclination to "experiment" with one's sexual preferences. Should you decide to experiment with your sexual preferences, make sure you are always honest with yourself and any potential partners.

Positions. In and out, up and down can get pretty boring after a while. Let's face it, the same old missionary position can become monotonous, so many people desire to liven things up by experimenting with positions. Kama Sutra is one of the most famous manuals that depict a variety of usual and unusual sexual positions with interesting names such as "The Glowing Universe." Talking about seeing stars! Although many of the positions require Olympic standard flexibility, the fun of it all is just trying new positions!

Ménage a trois. Proceed with extreme caution! The thought of inviting a third person into your sex play might sound like a great idea, but there are some things to consider before "experimenting" with a ménage. It's definitely not for the faint at heart! Honesty, trust, communication and caution are just a few things that will help keep this dream from turning into a nightmare. Including a third person between the sheets must be something that all parties willingly negotiate, agree to and are involved in throughout the entire process. If one person in the trio becomes uncomfortable, then do not continue until all parties involved are comfortable and in agreement. No one should be coerced or tricked into participating in a "threesome." It is important to keep in mind that having a ménage a trois will not solidify or repair a troubled relationship. In most cases, it will have the exact opposite effect and ultimately cause more harm to your relationship. Also, if either you or your partners are prone to jealousy, then a ménage is NOT for you.

Role play. A role play can be a fun and flirty way to add some excitement to your sexual script! Create the fantasy and act it out! You are only limited by your imagination. Experiment with a variety of costumes, scenarios and locations. A naughty school girl outfit can make the boring house wife or busy career woman seem like a brand new woman to her Beloved. FYI, can get in to character too! The handyman always fixes a thing or two and the pizza delivery guy knows exactly what to deliver!

Sex Toys. Who says toys are just for kids? There is a billion dollar industry devoted to creating toys just for adults! From vibrators to dildos, anal beads to sex swings and machines, experimenting with sex toys can be just what the doctor ordered to help spice up your sex life. With so many adult novelties on the market, one could literally create the playground of their dreams! If you want to get really creative, you can actually make your own sex toys by using common items found around your house. For example, that old hairbrush in your bathroom drawer can now become a whip to tame your lover.

So you're ready to spice up your sex life and you're not quite sure how to talk with your lover about including sex toys into your sex play? Sex toys can definitely break the monotony of the same old boring sex by adding flavor and excitement. However, introducing this third party to your partner and getting them to agree to incorporate them into your sex play can be a tricky task (but a very rewarding treat)!

Creating the union between your lover and your sex toy requires a very delicate balance between preserving your lover's ego and meeting your needs. You must choose your words wisely; one slip of the wrong word can result in certain disaster. You must make sure that your lover does not see the sex toy as his or her replacement, but rather, as an additional vehicle to ecstasy and fulfillment for both of you.

The following steps can help aid your transition into introducing the joys of sex toys into your lover's repertoire.

* Become a Sexpert on sex toys! Educate yourself on all the ins and outs of sex toys. You may want to pick up a copy of *Sex Toys 101* by Rachel Venning and Claire Cavanah. It's a playful, uninhibited, easy read with vivid imagery. Be sure to highlight all the benefits of incorporating sex toys into your sex play (increasing orgasmic intensity, variety, extra stimulation, etc.) You also may consider reading the book with your lover. Attending an adult novelty party like those that are sponsored by Pure Romance can be educational, fun and sexy as well.

- Choose an appropriate time to have THE conversation. This conversation must definitely take place before engaging in any sex play. Never try to surprise your lover with a sex toy during the act, as this may ruin the mood and you may find yourself in a very awkward position and/or the middle of a heated disagreement. Find out your lover's concerns regarding sex toys. Acknowledge and validate their feelings by assuring them that a sex toy can never replace the human bonding, intimacy and touch. In addition, sharing your sexual fantasies helps to build intimacy between you and your lover. It is also helps to keep love alive!

- Take a trip to an adult novelty store together. Turn the experience into an intimate journey into bliss. Look, touch and try the display models in the store. This can actually help build anticipation and excitement for what's to come or cum. Encourage your lover to select a toy that can be used on him or her and one that can be used on you. If you or your lover is a novice user, you may want to start with something basic. Read my article on How to choose a sex toy before going to the store, as this may help to alleviate some anxiety.

- Enjoy! Incorporating sex toys can open up a whole new and intriguing world. It can also help to breathe life into an otherwise dulling sex life.

With so many sex toys available, it can be difficult to choose one that's right for you. Where does one begin? Whether you're a sex toy enthusiast or novice, the important thing to remember when choosing a toy is your purpose for buying it. For the more seasoned sex toy aficionado, this may be an easy task. However, if you are just beginning to dabble with the joys of sex toys, you may want to start off with something a little less intimidating and work your way up. Shopping for the perfect sex toy can be overwhelming; to help ease any anxiety; you may consider talking with a sex coach or counselor, asking a romance specialist at an adult novelty store for assistance, or taking an educational sex toy workshop. Taking time to educate yourself about the various sex toys on the market and their uses will ultimately enhance your sexual pleasure and your life! To help you begin "Operation Sex Toy", here are some helpful tips to consider:

> *Intended Use: Who will be using the toy: alone or with a lover?*
> *Function: What do you want the toy to do for you: vibrate, rotate, twist? Does it need to be waterproof? What scenarios do you envision: bondage, power-play, sensory deprivation?*
> *Styles: What do you want the toy to look like? Modern, traditional, discreet?*
> *Material: What type of material do you like most: jelly, rubber, cyberskin, silicone, glass, metal, leather?*
> *Texture: Do you want smooth, ridges, studded, stones, encrusted, etc?*
> *Size: What size do you want—normal, small, large, pocket? You may also consider the width, length and shape.*
> *Prices: low or high end? Keep in mind, you get what you pay for!*

* Use a lubricant. Water- and silicone-based lubricants are safe to use with sex toys. Avoid using oil-based or petroleum-based lubricants as they break down latex material. Oil-based lubricants are for external use only and are great for massaging but not for using with a sex toy. In addition since the body does not properly breakdown oil-based lubricants, this increases the chances for infections. Also, be aware of lubricants that contain glycerin i.e. flavored lubricants, as this increases the potential for yeast infections in women. Using a lubricant is also important because it helps to serve as an extra protective barrier for the vagina which reduces the amount of tearing to the lining of the vagina; which also reduces risk of transmission of bacteria, virus, etc. Remember the wetter the better!

- Clean your sex toy. Since sex toys are used on the most sensitive parts of your body, it makes sense to keep it well cleaned and cared for. With a few simple steps, you can prolong the life of your toy. Non-porous materials are smooth and warm water and soap usually does the trick. If needed, silicone sex toys can be sterilized by boiling it for 3 to 5 minutes. Porous materials such as cyberskin and rubber require a bit more care as bacteria can hide within the pores. Avoid using soap on cyberskin to maintain the texture. Instead, rinse with lots of warm water or sterilize with alcohol. It is best air-dried and sprinkled with cornstarch or talcum to maintain the smooth surface. To keep all your toys clean and ready to use, you can also pick up a "care & cleaning kit."

Storing Your Sex Toy

- Try to store sex toys within reach of the bed. Nothing is more frustrating than interrupting foreplay and having to walk across the room to dig out the toy from a secret hidden spot. Sex toys should be stored in protective casing or wrapped individually in a piece of cloth, away from prying eyes. There are several novelty items available such as the "Hide Your Vibe" pillow to discreetly store our sex toys, or you and your Beloved can have fun using your creativity to make your own "sex toy box."
- Safer Sex Tip: Use a condom. Condoms can be used with sex toys so that it reduces the risk of transmitted infections. Using a condom also makes it safer for sharing between partners and/or for use with multiple partners.
- Take with you an imagination as you enter the wonderful world of sex toys! Turn your experience into an adventurous treasure hunt as you discover the various sex toys on the market! Continue your hunt, exploring each and every device of sexual

pleasure until you find the one or the few that you enjoy the most! Unleash your inhibitions and let the journey begin!

Kink. *50 Shades of Grey* introduced "kinky sex" to the masses and now it has become mainstream, making it the "in thing." Flocks of people are rushing out to their local adult novelty store to pick up a grey tie, a pair of hair cuffs and a crop in an effort to imitate the infamous Christian Grey. However, before you go all in on the great BDSM experiment, it is very important that you understand the rules of "play" and have a safe word and/or signal just in case things become too intense. Remember the golden rule when it comes to kink is to keep it safe, sane and consensual. Never engage in any BDSM activities with someone that you have not established a trusting relationship with.

Sensory deprivation. Blindfold, tie me up and gag me! Take away one of the senses and the others will heighten. Falling under the umbrella of kink, sensory deprivation is a way to increase sexual arousal and intensify the orgasmic experience by depriving one or more of the senses. Warning! You must be very careful when "experimenting" with sensory deprivation because you could really hurt yourself or someone else, especially in the case of erotic asphyxiation. Sensory deprivation is not for everyone so before you begin restraining or pouring hot candle wax on your Beloved, you should definitely have a conversation with him or her. The use of a safe word or signal is important in any sensory deprivation play.

Scheduling sex. There's a myth that spontaneity is the hallmark of a good sexual relationship. While spontaneous sex can be lots of fun, life rarely affords us the opportunity for perfect circumstances or opportunity for sex, so why spend your life waiting for a moment that may never come. Sometimes you just have to schedule time for sex. I know what you're thinking — schedule time for sex? Absolutely! We take to schedule or nail appointments, hair appointments, doctors' appointments, weddings, vacations and any other thing that is of importance to us, right? So if sex is important, then take the time to schedule it. If you are concern about the spontaneity of things, do not be. Just because you make an appointment does not mean you know exactly what to expect sexually, and that is where the spontaneity comes in. Spontaneity also comes in with the positions and location.

Sex beyond the bedroom. Location! Location! Location! is everything when it comes to sex. Whether it is in the car, on the kitchen table, in a grassy field, on the beach, in the shower or on the living room floor, moving beyond the bedroom can definitely spice things up. Your sex life may be doing alright, with the same positions and the same place every time, but there is always room for improvement! Variety is the spice of LIFE! It is time to change that old boring sex script, break the monotony and try some fun and unusual places beyond your bedroom.

Quickies. Don't allow your sex life to become a "maybe" or "if I get around to it!" What better way to get the momentum going again than with a quickie? A quickie is an excellent way to connect with your Beloved while boosting your libido and saying goodbye to the dreadful sex rut. Rip each other's clothes off! Don't' worry about how your hair or body looks! Moan loudly! Breathe deeply! Hold each other tightly like your lives depend on it! Most of all live in the moment! Carpe Diem!

Non-penetrative/Non-Sexual Activities. Consider doing some non-sexual or non-penetrative/intercourse activities that will help to increase the intimate connection between the two of you. Such activities include: dancing, sensual massage, breathing exercises, cuddling naked, showering together, yoga, reading erotica together, play lover's games, etc.

"Sexperimenting" can be extremely fun, but just how far you decide to take it is really up to you (and your partner). You can choose to jump right in or just simply ease your way into the "sex lab." Whatever you decide, it is important to always be open and honest with yourself and others as this will help to minimize risk of injury and hurt to all involved. If all things have been considered, discussed and agreed upon then you are all ready to go! Get your sexual pleasure!

"My Beloved, you have found your sexual voice!"

You may wonder why I chose to make sexual pleasure the last section of the book. While sexual pleasure is an important component of sexuality, it should not be the focus! Our sexuality is so much more than pleasure or intercourse! It's who we are and who we were created to be! We must honor and respect our sexuality at all times!

Now that you have found your sexual voice, it is your responsibility to share! You are charged with sharing this valuable L.I.F.E.-changing and L.I.F.E.-saving information with your daughters, sisters, aunts, sister friends, mothers and even grandmothers. We must keep this message of healthy sexuality moving! When we share this message of healthy sexuality, we leave a lasting legacy that empowers a generation to make sustainable behavior changes that will forever change the trajectory of women's sexuality in a powerful way!

It is time for women to create a new sexual blueprint and reclaim our sexual images, not just our own but for society as well. We must ask ourselves several questions:

* Is our sexual integrity worth protecting?
* Do we care about the type of image our girls see growing up?
* Is their public image worth defending?
* How do we break these unhealthy and negative images of our sexuality?

We certainly have a responsibility to ourselves and future generations of women. No longer can we remain silent, or stand idly on the sidelines while the images of our sexuality continue to be destroyed in society. In order to change the trajectory, we need to begin with restoring women's sense of value, worth and sexuality. Once we do, we will be to see a shift in our society that will begin to embrace and celebrate women's sexuality!

Dr. TaMara Griffin Bio

DR. TAMARA LOVES NOTHING MORE than talking about sex! At the age of 13, she told her mother she wanted to be a Sex Therapist! Her passion is deeply rooted in spreading messages about healthy sexuality. Dr. TaMara is a certified clinical sexologist, sex therapist, best selling author and powerful motivational speaker with more than 20 years of experience speaking, writing and teaching about sexuality. She travels the country helping individuals embrace and honor their sexuality. Dr. TaMara has published numerous books and articles. She is the owner of L.I.F.E. by Dr. TaMara- Live Inspired Feel Empowered LLC-LIFE. Dr. TaMara is also the Editor-in-Chief of Our Sexuality! Magazine. Our Sexuality! is the premiere magazine for women's sexuality and sexual health. Dr. TaMara is the National Correspondent and a "Thought Leader" for the Association of Black Sexologist and Clinicians. She is also a member of the American College of Sexologists International. Follow her on Twitter, Facebook at LIFE by Dr. TaMara or Instagram, or her Live Inspired Feel Empowered (L.I.F.E.) blog www.drtamaragriffin. com. Join Dr. TaMara movement of Healthy Sexuality **#HowDareINot #ISaveLives** www.howdareinot.com

Appendix A

I Love SEX Quiz Answers.

ARE THESE STATEMENTS TRUE OR FALSE?

1. Sexual intercourse is the first sexual activity for females. **False**
2. Self-Pleasure has always been recognized as normal sexual behavior. **False**
3. All orgasms are the same. **False**
4. Exercising can increase sexual pleasure and orgasmic intensity. **True**
5. 95% of women DO NOT experience orgasm through self-pleasure. **False**
6. The majority of women need direct clitoral stimulation to reach orgasm. **True**
7. Self-Pleasure is often prescribed for pre-orgasmic women. **True**
8. Stimulating the G-spot can cause female ejaculation. **True**
9. The clitoris is made of erectile tissue. **True**
10. There is a difference between arousal and desire. **True**
11. Vibrators were first prescribed to treat hysteria in women. **True**
12. Body image and sexuality are closely related. **True**
13. Self-esteem and sexuality are closely related. **True**
14. Women can experience a variety of different types of orgasms. **True**
15. Unlike men, women DO NOT experience a refractory period. **True**